Advance Pr

"Barbara Rodge...
pensable and urgently vital book dealing
with the future of mankind! The alarm-
ing increase in infertility and autistic
spectrum disorder in our modern com-
puterized age has been the harbinger of
tragic outcomes for many growing families. This significant and timely book
reveals a safe, simple and strategic protocol for young women preparing for conception. Rodgers offers tremendous hope
and easily workable nutritional solutions
for couples in the 21st Century. This is a
must-read book as infertility and autistic
spectrum disorder literally touches us all."

Stephen Sinatra, M.D., F.A.C.C.,
F.A.C.N. Co-author, *Health
Revelations from Heaven and Earth*

"Barbara's book is a breath of fresh air. I
have always said that the biggest impact
we can have on the health of the planet
is to assist in the conception and raising
of healthy babies. Barbara lays out the
proper steps needed for moms, and dads,
to position themselves in conceiving and
birthing the healthiest and happiest child
possible. Thank you for this powerful
book, written in a very easy and understandable fashion for all. For all you par-

ents out there. You can't say there isn't an owners' manual any more, Barbara created this for you right here. Enjoy!"

Glen Depke, Traditional Naturopath
Speaker, Author, Trainer
and Founder of Depke Wellness
DepkeWellness.com

"*Baby Maker* is a breath of fresh, much-needed air in a world where couples, desperate to have a baby, are pushed toward expensive, high-tech solutions to 'unexplained' infertility. Barbara Rodgers has done her homework. She explains what fertility doctors often overlook—the environmental factors, particularly nutrition, that are lowering fertility rates around the world. After laying out the scientific research on the "Why?" of infertility, she goes on to share concrete actions for becoming fertile and raising healthy babies. *Baby Maker* is a must-read for women contemplating making babies."

Tom Ballard, RN, ND
Founder: Natural DNA Solutions
Author of Nutrition-1-2-3 and
Genetic Health Reports, as well as the
natural medicine mystery novel, *The Last Quack* (fun with food and feathers!)
www.PureWellnessCenters.com

"*Baby Maker* is an excellent overview of what to do to help ensure the healthiest pregnancy, as well as setting up baby and parents for a lifetime of wellness. So often the act of becoming pregnant and carrying to term is the whole intent of parents-to-be and their providers, but *Baby Maker* gives the tools necessary for not only increased chances of fertility for both parents, but also sets the stage so that the parents will be in robust health throughout the pregnancy and in the best condition to look after their new child after the pregnancy and delivery (and as all parents know, middle-of-the-night feedings, recovery from birth, a healthy and replete milk supply for nursing, and adjusting to the all-encompassing responsibilities of continued care for a newborn are monumental and completely engrossing tasks!) This book should be required reading for anyone looking to start a family—as well as their doctors and health care providers!"

Dr. Sarica Cernohous, L.Ac.
Author of *The Funky Kitchen: Easy Techniques from Our Ancestors for Improved Digestion, Enhanced Vitality and Joy!*

"*Baby Maker* is the perfect resource for couples preparing for pregnancy. Barbara Rodgers gives compelling reasons for wanna-be moms and dads to adopt a healthy lifestyle well in advance of conception. She lays out an easy-to-follow, step-by-step plan for improving health (men and women) to support fertility, conception, as well as recommendations to maintain health during mom's pregnancy, breastfeeding and post-delivery—it is truly an A to Z manual for making healthy babies!"

Miriam Zacharias – MS, NTC, BCHN
Author, *The PEACE Process*

"Barbara Rodgers has provided a much-needed resource for what has become a minefield of toxicity, trauma, and tears. I remember how devastated I was when I read that human breast milk had become one of the most toxic substances on the planet. I realized then that couples had to be very intentional in their plans for conception if they wanted a healthy baby. This book is just what the doctor ordered! If you plan to have a baby, know someone who plans on having a baby, or want to give the best baby shower gift ever, get this book."

Dr. Keesha Ewers, #1 bestselling
author of *Solving the Autoimmune Puzzle* and *The Quick and Easy Autoimmune Paleo Cookbook*

"Finally, we have a plan that makes sense for young couples who want to start a family! In *Baby Maker*, Barbara Rodgers has provided future parents a roadmap of how to improve fertility, have a healthy pregnancy, and deliver happy, healthy babies into their waiting arms—all based on holistic nutrition and natural health protocols. This book belongs in the hands of every couple who dream of becoming parents one day."

Patricia Koss, PhD, NC, FNLP – www.getnourishedpdx.com

"Joy to the world, a much-needed book has finally been written that addresses the science of fertility with clear explanations for the continual rise of infertility we are experiencing. Barbara Rodgers presents us with wise, compassionate solutions, offering a path to healthy pregnancy and birth. We can celebrate the birth of this book that will support healthy babies and provide great delight for parents who have not found their way to such a nutritious journey to success. Bravo...a must read."

Paula Bartholomy, CNC, BCHN, Registrar and Director of Online Events at Hawthorn University https://www.hawthornuniversity.org/

"I sure could have used this book before, during and after my VERY rocky pregnancy! While I was able to get pregnant with my son, I wasn't able to conceive a second time. My one pregnancy was fraught with challenges. I had morning sickness that stayed with me until the day I delivered, I gained nearly 50 pounds, and my mood swings were more dramatic than any other time in my life. My desire to breastfeed my beautiful baby boy became a nightmare, when my milk didn't come in properly. The doctor repeatedly (and rather frustratedly!) tried to assure me that, "every mother makes the right amount of milk for her baby." He couldn't have been more wrong; my son was STARVING! Eventually and much earlier than I wanted, I abandoned breastfeeding altogether.

"This book could have changed all of that for me and my baby. Barb has done her research and provides a treasure-trove of specific information that will help you avoid so many of the problems I encountered. Having an education in Holistic Nutrition now myself, I know that so much of what I experienced was because my diet was lacking. Getting the right nutrients through food and supplements could have made my pregnancy more enjoyable, helped my milk come in properly, and might have set the stage for my dream of having a second child.

"There's nothing more amazing than holding your baby in your arms for the first time. When you look into your baby's eyes, you'll want to feel confident that you did all you could to give him the best start in life. If you want to have the healthiest pregnancy possible, read this book and follow Barb's advice."

Nicole Hodson, NC, BCHN™
Executive Director, National Association
of Nutrition Professionals (NANP)

"Throughout history, cultures have taken great effort to nourish individuals in preparation for conception and child rearing. Today we call it pre-conception planning or nourishment, a long over-looked process that ensures a successful pregnancy, as well as healthy, happy children to build the future. At last here is a grounded well-researched approach to preconception-nourishment and well mother and baby nutrition care. With today's modern rush and abundance of manufactured foods combined with medications women and especially those who are pregnant do not 'appreciate that, biochemically, the odds are stacked against them.' This single sentence jumped off the page when I read *Baby Maker*, and a new understanding resulted. As an instructor to Holistic Nutrition students, this understanding gained from reading Barbara Rodgers, *Baby Maker*, will help me in educating the next generation on the importance of 'stacking the deck for success' for mother and baby alike."

Tammera J. Karr, Ph.D., BCHN,
Author of *Our Journey with Food*

BABY MAKER

A Complete Guide to Holistic Nutrition for Fertility, Conception, and Pregnancy

BARBARA RODGERS, NC, BCHN

Post Hill
PRESS

A POST HILL PRESS BOOK

ISBN: 978-1-68261-734-2
ISBN (eBook): 978-1-68261-735-9

Baby Maker:
A Complete Guide to Holistic Nutrition for
Fertility, Conception, and Pregnancy

This book contains advice and information relating to healthcare. It should be used to supplement rather than replace the advice of your doctor or another trained health professional. If you know or suspect that you have a health problem, it is recommended that you seek your physician's advice before embarking on any medical program or treatment. All efforts have been made to assure the accuracy of the information in this book as of the date of publication. The publisher and the author disclaim liability for any medical outcomes that may occur as a result of applying the methods suggested in this book.

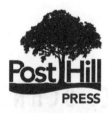

Post Hill Press, LLC
New York • Nashville
posthillpress.com

Published in the United States of America

DEDICATION

*To my dear friend and trusted mentor, Ann Boroch, who trag-
ically left this planet far too soon. You encouraged, motivated,
and inspired me to write this book and to use my own healing
experience with Holistic Nutrition to help others. From your
place among the angels, I hope you know how much you are
loved and missed.*

*Lastly, this book is dedicated to all the loving, conscientious
men and women who already cherish the new life that is waiting
to become part of theirs.*

Before you were conceived,
I wanted you....

Before you were born,
I loved you....

Before you were here an hour,
I knew I would do anything for you.

Children are the miracle of life.

—Unknown Author

CONTENTS

Important Notice to the Reader 11

How to Use This Book 13

Foreword...15

Introduction 19

Chapter 1—Looking for Baby in All the Wrong Places:
  Planning for Success...27
    Planning for All the Wrong Things......................31
    Is Poor Nutrition Linked to Infertility?................32
    What's in Your Genes?.......................................33
    Healthy Takes Center Stage 39
    Whom and What Do You Believe? 40
    Waking Up to the Positive Impact of Nutrition...42
    Strategic Pregnancy-Planning—
        Nutrition Matters..44
Chapter 2—How to Find Fertility: Causes, Signs,
  Symptoms, and Tracking.......................................45
    Understanding Unexplained Infertility 46
    Is Your Current Diet Enhancing Fertility or
        Damaging It?..49
    Causes of Infertility in Women..........................51

Health Conditions and Diseases That May
   Cause Female Infertility.................................. 52
Causes of Infertility in Men................................. 53
Diagnostic Testing and Tracking
   Signs of Fertility... 57
Self-Testing for Fertility and Ovulation 58
Tech-Savvy Methods of Tracking Fertility............ 60
Traditional Fertility-Tracking Methods................ 61
Other Signs of Ovulation and Fertility 63

**Chapter 3—You and Your Baby Are Bugged: Your
Microbiome and How It Affects Fertility.................65**
What Is the Human Microbiome?...................... 67
Where Are the Bacteria?.................................... 69
The Role Microbes Play in the Human Body
   and How to Protect Them 71
Why You Need to Be Bugged to Have a
   Healthy Pregnancy.. 76
Mom's Bugs, Pregnancy, and Baby...................... 77
Childbirth and Seeding Your Baby's
   Microbiome 78
Your Microbiome and Breastfeeding.................... 80

**Chapter 4—Eating the Baby-Maker Way: What to
Eat to Have a Healthy Pregnancy 83**
A Healthy Pregnancy Introduction 84
"My Pregnancy Plate".. 86
Food Nuances 89
Let's Talk about Weight Gain 91
Food Cravings.. 94
Blood Sugar, Glycemic Index, and
   Gestational Diabetes...................................... 96
Healthy Eating by Food Group 106
Summary of Dietary Recommendations
   during Pregnancy 136

Summary of Foods to Avoid during Pregnancy.. 139
Get Yourself Organized..................................... 144

Chapter 5—The Baby-Maker Strategy: Your Strategies for Fertility, Pre-Conception, and Pregnancy 146
Pre-Conception Strategy for Women 147
Eleven Key Steps to Fertility—Women.............. 149
Pre-Conception Strategy for Men—
    Ten Key Steps for Fertility 158
Nutrition and Lifestyle Strategy during
    Pregnancy.. 166
Summary of Foods to Avoid during Pregnancy.. 172
Supplement Recommendations for
    Pre-Conception and Pregnancy 177
Nutrient Requirements during Breastfeeding..... 181

Chapter 6—Eating the Baby-Maker Way by Trimester: What to Eat to Have a Healthy Pregnancy by Trimester 184
Pregnancy Changes Everything......................... 186
Eating Healthy—First Trimester....................... 187
Eating Healthier—Second Trimester 193
Still Eating Healthy—Third Trimester............... 196

Chapter 7—Don't Mess with Your Hormones: Important Things to Avoid during Pre-conception and Pregnancy...202
Foods to Avoid 203
Lifestyle Issues to Avoid................................... 206

Chapter 8—Healthy Mom, Happy Baby: Recommendations for Post-Pregnancy Diet and Health 215
Bringing Home Baby—A Reality Check 216
Getting Back to Normal—Don't Rush It.......... 219
Early Days after Delivery................................... 220

Up to Six Weeks after Delivery............................ 222
Seven Weeks to Four Months after Delivery or Post-
    Breastfeeding.. 224
Four Months to One Year after Delivery............. 226
One to Two Years following Delivery.................. 228
Two Years and Later following Delivery.............. 229
Postpartum Depression 230
Breastfeeding: Nutritional Guidelines................ 232
The Formula-Fed Infant 248
Sleep-Deprivation.. 249
Chapter 9—Not All Supplements Are Created Equal:
Choose and Buy Supplements like a Pro 253
Why Take Supplements?..................................... 254
Everyone Is Nutrient-Deficient........................... 256
Is Your Food "Healthy"? 257
Who Is Paying Attention to Supplement
    Manufacturers?.. 258
Don't Waste Your Money—Buy Quality............. 260
Where to Buy Supplements................................ 265
Appendix 269
Bone Broth Recipe 269
Food Sources of Potassium 273
Baby-Maker Fertility and Pregnancy Smoothie.. 274
Summary of Foods to Avoid during Pregnancy.. 277
Pre-Conception Detoxification Instructions 283
Detoxifying Green Drink Recipe........................ 287
Antioxidant Salad Recipe................................... 289
List of Cruciferous Vegetables............................ 291
Sources of Gluten.. 292
Summary of Daily Recommended
    Food Servings.. 298

Endnotes..303
Acknowledgments...323
About the Author...325

IMPORTANT NOTICE TO THE READER

This book contains nutritional and lifestyle information that is available in the public domain and is presented strictly for informational and educational use only. This information is not intended as medical advice, nor should any portion of it be considered as diagnosing, treating, preventing, or curing any disease or health condition.

The author realizes that the treatment of any health condition and the enhancement of health through nutritional changes should be supervised by a qualified, licensed healthcare practitioner, and only those licensed can legally offer medical advice in the United States. Consult your doctor before starting any of the recommendations suggested here. This book will be especially complemented by discussions with a physician or other licensed provider who has training or expertise in nutrition.

The author and publisher do not assume medical or legal liability for personal loss caused or alleged to be caused, directly or indirectly, through the use or misuse of the information or recommendations contained in this book.

HOW TO USE THIS BOOK

Although the information contained in this book is based on research and science, I have attempted to use language that makes the concepts presented easy to understand. For the sake of brevity, and to accommodate the non-medical or non-science reader, some concepts are described in a manner that provides you with a broad overview only, which avoids some of the science jargon and in-depth descriptions that would turn this book into several volumes of material.

Although each chapter contains important information about supporting health for men and women from the early stage of only considering pregnancy to the first several weeks after delivery, you have the option of using it as a reference tool, going back and forth to chapters that contain information that will be useful for you based on where you are on this spectrum. I hope the majority of you will read it cover to cover, but I think you will find it a useful resource without doing so.

I would also like to clarify references made throughout the book to "moms and dads," "women and men," and so forth. These references are used for simplicity's sake and are not meant to exclude those who do not meet the traditional definition of a "man," "woman," or "couple." I am aware and supportive of the transgender, gay, and lesbian communities who may not fall into these traditional roles but who, in fact, share the traditional values, hopes, and dreams of giving birth.

FOREWORD

I really loved the title of this book! I was just as impressed with the content that covered such current and urgent topics as fertility, conception, and pregnancy for so many women and their partners.

As a *New York Times* multi-award-winning author, researcher, and woman's health advocate, I can say that this seminal book you are holding in your hands is the most integrative guide to "baby making" I have reviewed in the past thirty years. Of the myriad of topics and requests for books that my readers have requested over the years, *Baby Maker* is the one that is most popular by far. So, not only is this book truly overdue, but it is also a most welcome literary resource for women, their families (especially their husbands), and care givers. It is a wonderful addition for physicians, nurses, naturopaths, chiropractors, health coaches, and nutritionists. And best of all for those with unresolved fertility issues and a history of miscarriages, this book offers hope.

The author of this labor of love, Barbara Rodgers, is eminently qualified to write about the topic of baby making as she has lived it. She has firsthand knowledge of the impact nutrition has on a woman's body from giving birth and raising two beautiful daughters as well as using nutrition to resolve severe symptoms of multiple sclerosis. Not only is she an expert in prenatal nutrition, but she is well versed in many other areas of healthcare, including the management of autoimmune conditions.

With hands-on knowledge and experience in the process of creating a new human being, this is the book that everyone has been waiting for. In my view, her awareness that we are living in a toxic day and age is fundamental to understanding the information that she presents. I believe a healthy body is a clean body. Yet, as we are moving through the 21st Century, this is becoming virtually unattainable. Toxins seem to be proliferating all around us, especially hormone disruptors. We find them in the food we eat, affecting the environment, and even impacting our body's metabolic processes. With a weakened immune system, some of us are becoming infertile too soon and older before our time—having major problems with conception, gaining weight, and becoming vulnerable to an entire host of hormone-induced and degenerative diseases.

The Baby Maker approach to fertility, conception, and pregnancy is quite timely.

Ms. Rodgers recognizes that it is no longer our mother or grandmother's world anymore. Navigating through the challenges of the environment and learning how to eat in each phase of pregnancy and thereafter is essential for a longer, more vigorous life and bringing a baby into our world.

I am very happy Barbara Rodgers wrote this book. Whether you are seeking to become pregnant, are already pregnant, or desire to have another child, the tools provided in this book will be extremely useful. This is the book I wish I could have written, but I am so thrilled and grateful we have *Baby Maker* for all of us now!

Ann Louise Gittleman, PhD, CNS,
NY Times Bestselling Author of 35 books

INTRODUCTION

"Infertility" Redefined

Everyone knows what to do to make a baby. A man and woman have unprotected sex...in most cases, often. Most couples go about starting their family with the glee, enthusiasm and naiveté of a child on their first day of kindergarten. They look forward to the fun and new experiences of having a child, but have no idea of the challenges that lay ahead, or the learning curve that must be tackled in order to achieve a successful pregnancy.

When a couple has been trying to conceive for three or four months, reality starts to sink in that this might not be as easy as they thought. Why isn't this just "happening"? Still confident in their natural ability to get pregnant, they begin research—a visit with her gynecologist, possibly a referral to a fertility specialist. Tests are ordered, period tracking commences, as does the escalating depression and worry that goes along with each new failed attempt at conception after having sex. None of that compares, however, to the blow that is administered when a couple hears the words "unexplained infertility."

About one in five couples are diagnosed with unexplained infertility.[1] In other words, there is no known medical reason that pregnancy cannot occur. Tests have not revealed poor egg quality. There are no obvious infections or physical abnormalities. While this technically is good news, it can also be very unsettling. Now these couples are faced with some big questions. What is preventing them from achieving pregnancy? What do they have to do to have a baby? Can they afford IUI (intrauterine insemination) or IVF (in vitro fertilization)? Is there a "cure" for infertility? I believe that in many cases there is, and there is plenty of science to back me up, upon which I have based the facts and recommendations in this book.

Surprise—You Have an Incurable Disease!

There are unexpected and powerful experiences that inspired me to write this book. No, I'm not going to bore you with my own dreadful tale of how horribly I ate during my pregnancies, how I gained fifty pounds during each, or how I genetically passed on insulin resistance to my daughters as a result of a high-sugar diet while pregnant.

Although all relevant and true, the first experience that set me off in the direction of this book had nothing to do with having babies. It had to do with a run-in I had with an incurable disease. My surprise diagnosis wasn't infertility; it was another type of a so-called incurable condition, an autoimmune disease.

As I completed my first year in my studies in Holistic Nutrition, I had also just completed my third year on the very restrictive "candida diet" to fight the debilitating symptoms of multiple sclerosis.

MS is a disabling autoimmune disease that disrupts communication within the nervous system.[2] Current statistics show that it affects an estimated two and a half million people around the world, nearly a half a million of them in the U.S.[3]

Unless you have an autoimmune condition, you probably aren't familiar with the specific diet protocols that make up a candida diet. It combines aspects of paleo, ketogenic, Mediterranean, and Atkins all rolled up into one big, seriously challenging diet. Let me tell you; it's not for the faint of heart, but it works.

During the years I dealt with MS, I learned firsthand how critical the health of the GI tract is to overall health, the horrible, debilitating effects of an impaired immune system, and the immense power that food has on the human body. The candida diet tackles all of this head-on by eliminating the types of food that cause an overgrowth of candida in the GI tract. In my case, that meant changing nearly my entire diet.

Through the years of my life up until that point, my normal diet would be described as "reverse Paleo." Or maybe a better label would be "anti-healthy." Pretty much everything I consumed was laced with sugar. Sugar and carbs are big no-no's on the candida diet, so I had to eliminate almost everything I loved to eat. It was extremely difficult to stay disciplined. I frequently used my debilitating and deteriorating physical condition as motivation to stick with the program. I was desperate to feel well again, to regain my stamina, and to feel stable and strong on my feet. I clung to anything that offered hope. My new diet was my hope. Nutritious, whole foods became symbols of healing. For you they will become symbols of fertility.

During those challenging three years on my dietary program I became very tuned in to my body. If I ate something that wasn't "allowed," my body let me know within 24 to 48 hours. In the early months, an infraction would result in an escalation of MS symptoms. In my case that meant tingling and numbness in my left foot, weakness in my lower extremities, and an almost unbearable exacerbation of fatigue, my primary symptom.

In the latter months of my diet, my body's reactions to the disallowed foods became less severe; my tolerance improved. I didn't understand back then, but the increase in tolerance was a clear indication that my immune system was also in better shape than when I started. The diet was working.

Most of us have heard the expression "You are what you eat." What I learned through my experiences with my own health issues was more accurately described by Ann Wigmore's quotation:

> *"The food you eat can either be the safest*
> *and most powerful form of medicine or the*
> *slowest form of poison."*
>
> —*Ann Wigmore*

As I regained functionality and energy in my body from the dietary changes I had made, it became crystal clear in my mind that the many years and decades prior to my MS diagnosis, I had been slowly poisoning myself. From my childhood well into adulthood, my diet consisted of sugary foods, carbohydrates (bad ones, not the good ones), lots of coffee and alcohol, junk food, fast food, and processed food. Pile on a high-stress corporate job with lots of travel, teenagers at home, long work hours, sleep-deprivation, tons of aspirin, Tylenol, and antibiotics for chronic infections, and the only thing more shocking than being diagnosed with multiple sclerosis was that it didn't cripple me years earlier.

Point made loud and clear: *Food Is Powerful.*

With a lot of hard work and dedication to my own health, I continued to climb out of the deep MS abyss. Today I have been symptom-free of an autoimmune response for a few years and consider myself cured. Yes, that's right...cured of an "incurable" disease. As you can imagine, my entire experience of getting healthy was uplifting, compelling, and life-changing. I wanted to learn more. And I did.

My traumatic health experience became my inspiration to begin a formal education in Holistic Nutrition. I became fascinated and intrigued at how nutrition, or more specifically, poor nutrition, affects the human body. As mentioned above, MS affects hundreds of thousands of people in the U.S. and instances of it are increasing[4]. On the other hand, infertility affects seven and a half million women between the ages of 15 and 44, and instances of it are also increasing.[5] Clearly there are enormous numbers of people who could benefit from learning more about the pervasive effects of poor nutrition.

In my studies I learned that the increasing rates of infertility in the U.S. may be directly linked to toxins and nutrient deficiencies to which we are subjecting our bodies. Furthermore, research indicates that women with unexplained infertility show significant dietary deficiencies when compared with fertile women.[6] Doesn't it make perfect sense that if a depleted, poorly nourished body could lead to my autoimmune disease, why not infertility in others?

By paying attention to diet and overall health a few months prior to any attempts to conceive, a man and woman could potentially save themselves from the heart-wrenching trauma of dealing with infertility, miscarriage, or an unhealthy pregnancy. Interesting, right? I was able to reclaim my health and my life by changing what I ate. Dietary changes (and sometimes lifestyle changes as well) have the potential to influence hormonal signaling, sperm counts, and ovum quality.[7]

The Bottom Line

My goal in writing this book is to help those who are pregnant or thinking of becoming pregnant understand that *nutrition matters*. Your health status prior to becoming pregnant *matters*. It determines how quickly you will get pregnant, helps maintain your health during pregnancy, and will greatly influence the health of your baby, as well as his or her genetic expression. What you eat and subject your body to every day sets the stage for optimal or deficient health status.

Baby Maker is packed with information that will help you improve your health status in order to achieve conception and have a healthy pregnancy. I share clear, easy-to-adopt options for improving fertility (for men and women), strengthening the ability of a pregnant mom to carry to term, and a plan to support the mom's health during pregnancy. I lay out supporting evidence as to why advanced planning is critical, specific recommendations and details on what steps need to be taken, as well as food lists and charts to help with meal-planning, food selection, and purchasing nutritional supplements. Finally, there is basic information offered on how to help get a new mom off to a good start immediately following delivery. I'm excited at the outcome I know you will have following the guidelines it lays out.

I want each soon-to-be-parent out there to be armed with credible, detailed, up-to-date information on how to get healthy and stay healthy before, during, and immediately following pregnancy. Just as I was able to reverse the course of a so-called incurable disease, changing how and what you eat will play a pivotal role in ensuring your fertility, a healthy pregnancy, healthy baby, and an elated, healthy mom and dad.

You have high hopes and dreams of being a loving, devoted mommy one day soon. Let your quest for fertility and a healthy pregnancy be your first step in responsible parenting.

You can do this, and I am honored to be a part of your journey.

CHAPTER 1

Looking for Baby in All the Wrong Places: Planning for Success

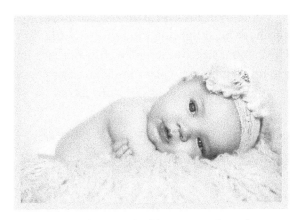

Source: © Photographed by Jamie Solorio | www. jamiesoloriophotography.com. Used with permission.

"Our goals can only be reached through a vehicle of a plan, in which we must fervently believe, and upon which we must vigorously act. There is no other route to success."

—Pablo Picasso

I know that you may be thinking that you don't want to have a "plan" for getting pregnant. We all know what we need to do to get pregnant, right? A man and a woman have unprotected sex and *voila*—let the pregnancy begin! However, you might be surprised to learn that it's just not that easy for most couples.

Bringing a new life into the world is the closest thing we know of to a real-life miracle. Developing a health strategy (or plan) for fertility and pregnancy doesn't sound very magical. And yet, there are tens of thousands of women every year who struggle with unexplained infertility, carrying a fetus to full term, or delivering a healthy child. While having a health strategy may be prosaic to some of you, it may also be the most viable, non-invasive path to becoming a parent for those who have been fighting the fertility battle. In Chapter 5 I will give you a step-by-step plan. But first, it's important for you to understand why planning is so critical, and why it will dramatically increase your odds of success.

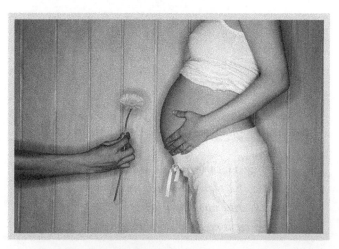

Source: Flickr.com, Jens Bergander, June 20, 2013

Let's first consider a hypothetical scenario.

Somewhere in the U.S. a woman in her early thirties has learned she is pregnant. As it happens with so many couples, this pregnancy was a welcome surprise. Neither she nor her husband did any planning for the pregnancy, but they are thrilled nonetheless and can't wait to start making arrangements to welcome their beautiful new baby into their lives.

Unfortunately, without any advanced planning, neither prospective parent had a chance to change his or her lifestyle or eating habits before conception. They are blissfully unaware of the health challenges they potentially face as a result.

Her daily life is filled with stress at work, a long commute, and a diet that takes advantage of the many conveniences American culture has to offer—fast, inexpensive food; frozen and packaged meals; lots of sugary carbohydrates and snacks; a constant need for the pick-me-up caffeine offers; minimal water for hydration; and few, if any, vegetables.

This soon-to-be mom is moderately overweight, takes a prescription drug to help her get to sleep and something in the morning for her frequent anxiety attacks, is prescribed antibiotics two to three times a year for chronic UTI and sinus infections, and often finds that a few glasses of wine at night after work helps take the edge off from her busy workday.

She doesn't appreciate that, biochemically, the odds were stacked against her that she would get pregnant at all due to the drag these annoying issues had on her fertility. She also lacks insight into her diminished chances of carrying her baby to full term and the detrimental effects these issues have on her long-term health, the development of her fetus, or eventually, the health of her baby.

And there's Dad. Like most people, this dad believes his involvement in the health of his fetus begins and ends with his sperm getting to the right place. If his "guys" can hit the bullseye, his job is done. However, new research says, "Not so fast." According to Professor Sarah Robertson at the Robinson Institute of the University of Adelaide, the entire makeup of a man's seminal fluid (not just sperm) has a great deal to do with influencing sperm quality, as well as the nutrient composition in the maternal blood that nourishes the embryo found prior to formation of the placenta.[1] It also influences the development of a fetus and has long-term effects on a child's health. So the fact that this dad regularly consumes above-average amounts of alcohol, has an uncontrollable sweet tooth that has led to insulin resistance and excessive weight gain, and has blood pressure and cholesterol levels through the roof—all of these contribute to "fetal programming."[2] In other words, through the poor health of his seminal fluid, Dad has contributed several unwelcomed genetic traits to his unborn child.

As well-intended as this young couple will be about doing everything right for their new child, glaring warning signs are being overlooked that their health may not adequately support the normal development of their fetus. With a little foresight, and perhaps some not-so-romantic planning, many of the future challenges with their pregnancy and health of their child could have been minimized, maybe even eliminated.

Now, that rather bleak-sounding scenario may have sent chills down your spine if you're reading this and already know you are pregnant. Don't panic and definitely do not put down this book feeling that you have missed the healthy baby boat. It's never too late to get back on track, nutritionally speaking.

It's also never too late to start delivering high-impact nutrients to the cells of your body. I am living proof that even so-called incurable diseases can be reversed, so trust me; this is worth your effort, no matter what stage you're at in starting your family.

Planning for All the Wrong Things

Deciding to conceive a child and discovering that you are pregnant are two of life's most emotional, moving, and gratifying experiences. Typically, this excitement is more pronounced for the woman who is or will be carrying the child, but overall, what your future holds and the changes that will occur in your life as a result of the decision to conceive is nothing short of life-altering. No exaggeration!

Everything you do, think, feel, plan, talk about, consider, or read becomes baby-centered from this point on. You'll both definitely feel as though you have "baby on the brain."

Soon, you will have countless decisions to make: finding a doctor and a birthing facility, deciding to breast- or bottle-feed, picking a name, pacifier or no pacifier, choosing between cloth and disposable diapers, selecting a décor for the nursery…you get the idea. But parenting excellence shouldn't begin with these choices. The single, most impactful action you can take that will affect your child for its entire life is for *you* to be healthy when you conceive. To accomplish that requires planning.

In this book, I will share viable options for improving your fertility, strengthening your ability to carry a pregnancy to term, and delivering a healthy baby—all based on current research and statistics. Let's first take a closer look at how nutrition might be connected to fertility.

Is Poor Nutrition Linked to Infertility?

Perhaps you picked up this book because you have concerns about your ability to conceive or to carry a pregnancy to term. You may have a family history of infertility or miscarriage, you or your partner may be facing health issues that may affect conception or pregnancy, or perhaps you've been trying to conceive with no luck. (Yet!)

You're not alone.

You don't have to search too hard to discover that fertility rates in the U.S. have fallen to a record low as of 2013 of 6.25 percent of births among women of childbearing age.[3] There are many factors contributing to this decline, including a drop in the number of women who are in their peak childbearing years (ages twenty to thirty-four) as well as an increase in the number of women who postpone having children.[4]

But there are other interesting correlations to the falling fertility rates that can be made to milestones in the U.S. food industry, all of which point to possible nutritional deficiencies as major contributing factors.

Interestingly, the general fertility rate among women between the ages of 15 and 44 took a sharp downturn around 1958–59 and has continued in a more-or-less downward trend since then.[5]

I realize that talking about trends from sixty-plus years ago will sound like ancient history to many of you, and in our fast-paced world, I suppose it is. But remember that genetics have an integral role to play here as well. If you are a prospective parent and your parents were malnourished, eating lots of sugar or processed foods, abused alcohol, tobacco or drugs, or struggled with obesity or other diseases, those issues were passed on to you genetically and must be taken into consideration. As they say, knowledge is power. The more you know about your genetic history, the better prepared you can be as you develop your nutrition strategy for pregnancy. The really good news here is that science is proving that our genes express themselves differently—that is to say, they can turn on or off—based on external factors being introduced, such as nutrition. To cut through the science-jargon, this means that it is very possible to "turn on" your fertility by changing what you eat.

Understanding changes in gene expression is called "epigenetics." How nutrition impacts our genes' ability to express health or disease is studied in a research area called "nutrigenomics." According to Doctor Nathaniel Mead with the Environmental Health Perspectives, "Nutrigenomics is the integration of genomic science with nutrition…. Nutrition modifies the extent to which different genes are expressed and thereby modulates whether individuals attain the potential established by their genetic background."[6]

The research being done in nutrigenomics is changing how we study health and disease. We're learning that nourishing food sources, as well as environmental and lifestyle factors, play a significant role in the human body's ability to sustain good health. What is even more exciting is that we have also learned that through healthy nutrition we can influence our genes in a way that helps us minimize the risk of disease and health conditions such as infertility.

What's in Your Genes?

Nutrition is directly linked to gene expression. In order to understand how your genes may have been altered from your parents and grandparents, we need to take that stroll down memory lane and understand the historical changes that have occurred in our eating habits and food supply. Below are just a few highlights.

- Use of shortening and vegetable oils loaded with omega-6 fats skyrocketed between 1950 and 1959 as replacements for quality saturated fats that are high in healthy omega-3 fatty acids. The widely used vegetable oils are typically found in processed and fast food.[7]

The hydrogenation process makes them highly concentrated in trans fats, which are linked to inflammatory conditions, obesity, and heart disease when consumed in excess. Research has shown that consuming trans fats can increase your risk of infertility by as much as 70 percent.[8] It should be noted that in 2015, the FDA recognized the health risks of using trans fats in food processing and banned food manufacturing from using them after 2018. One small step in the right direction.

- Also related to the use of hydrogenated oils, people began replacing high-quality butter with margarine laden with trans fats in the early 1950s. Use of butter dropped sharply as the use of margarine simultaneously increased.

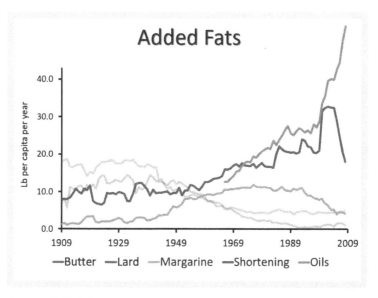

Source: USDA Economic Research Service, CDC NHANES Surveys, prepared by Doctor Stephan Guyenet, 2015, Whole Health Source Blog. As cited by Gunnars, K., Authority Nutrition, 2016.[9]

The irony here is that good-quality butter from grass-fed cows actually contains nutrients (such as vitamin K) that provide *protection* against inflammatory conditions and disease.[10]

- Per capita consumption of sucrose (i.e., sugar) in the U.S. skyrocketed around 1930 to eighty-five pounds per person. *The Washington Post* reported in February 2015 that the U.S. is the largest consumer of sugar in the world at more than 126 grams of sugar per person per day.[11] And guess what some of the negative effects of sugar are on the human body? Insulin resistance, lowered immunity, dysmenorrhea (severe PMS), yeast infections, and hormone disruption, to name a few. Having just one of those conditions can cause infertility.

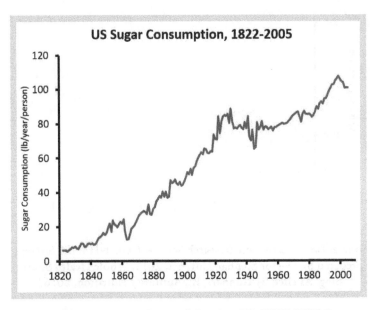

Source: USDA Economic Research Service, CDC NHANES Surveys, prepared by Doctor Stephan Guyenet, 2015, Whole Health Source Blog. As cited by Gunnars, K., Authority Nutrition, 2016.[12]

- Consumption of soda and fruit juice has increased sharply since the late 1970s. Some consider sugar-sweetened beverages one of the most damaging sources of sugar in our diet because they dramatically increase total caloric intake. These sugary beverages are directly correlated to obesity, weight gain, and incidence of diabetes.[13]

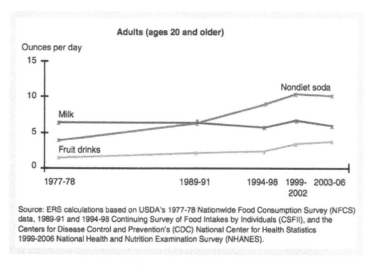

Adults (ages 20 and older)

Source: ERS calculations based on USDA's 1977-78 Nationwide Food Consumption Survey (NFCS) data, 1989-91 and 1994-98 Continuing Survey of Food Intakes by Individuals (CSFII), and the Centers for Disease Control and Prevention's (CDC) National Center for Health Statistics 1999-2006 National Health and Nutrition Examination Survey (NHANES).

Source: Centers for Disease Control and Prevention (CDC) National Center for Health Statistics 1992–2006 National Health and Nutrition Examination Survey (NHANES). As cited by Kris Gunnars, Healthline.com[14]

- Calorie intake in the U.S. has gone up 20 percent between 1970 and 2010. This is likely due to the consumption of processed foods, sugar consumption, increased food availability, as well as increased marketing directed to children.

- Consumption of processed foods and fast foods has escalated sharply since the early 1950s. Back in the olden days of the late 1800s, 93 percent of food was consumed at home and homemade from scratch. In 2009 barely half (51 percent) of food was consumed at home, and the rest was from full-service or fast food restaurants, which means for most of us, at least 50 percent of our food sources contain chemicals, toxins, trans fats, and sugar.

- Use of prescription medications rose dramatically starting in the 1950s with the development of new medicines, tranquilizers, amphetamines, opioids, weight-loss products, and over-the-counter pain-relievers such as Tylenol.[15] In spite of self-proclaimed success from the pharmaceutical manufacturers, male patients who discontinued medications, including antibiotics, for certain chronic diseases experienced an improvement in semen quality in 93 percent of participants and an 85 percent improvement in conception rates.[16]

- The rise of obesity in the U.S. began around the mid-1970s and directly correlates to USDA guidelines for a low-fat diet.

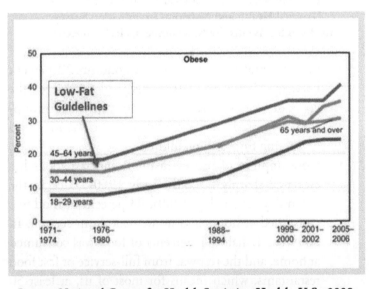

Source: National Center for Health Statistics. Health, U.S., 2008: With Special Feature on the Health of Young Adults. Hyattsville (MD): National Center for Health Statistics (US); 2009 Mar. Chartbook. As cited by Gunnars, K., Authority Nutrition, 2016.[17]

- Between 1954 and 1960 the FDA enacted some of the first legislation that allowed the use of food additives, pesticides, and color additives.[18] These substances are known as excitotoxins and endocrine disruptors—very fancy words for nasty little molecules that have the ability to kill off brain neurons, mess with blood sugar levels, disrupt hormone production and fertility, and increase production of free radicals leading to inflammation in the body.[19] The devastation they cause doesn't stop with fertility, unfortunately. Research on excitotoxins has broadened to suspected involvement in devastating diseases such as ALS, Parkinson's, and Alzheimer's disease.[20]

Chronic disease in the U.S. also began to escalate during the 1950s, including Alzheimer's disease, obesity, celiac, various cancers, diabetes, cardiovascular disease, and autoimmune disorders. Celiac disease has quintupled between the 1950s and 1990s.[21] Atherosclerosis (heart disease) is predicted to become the primary cause of death in the world by 2020.[22] And as cited earlier, fertility rates in the U.S. have continued to slowly decline during this same time period.

Healthy Takes Center Stage

Unfortunately, the commitment to health from most soon-to-be parents is often limited to making sure we take our prenatal vitamins regularly, occasionally eating some of the foods on the healthy food list we receive from our obstetrician, and of course, regularly monitoring weight gain. Consuming nutrient-dense foods just isn't on the radar, which seems strange to those of us who understand the basic principal of:

Garbage in = Garbage out

Or put another way:

Poor diet = Poor health

Or put yet another, more compelling way:

Poor parent health = Poor hormones, genetics, and baby health

If you really think about it, isn't it just a little arrogant to think you can eat a Dunkin' Donuts breakfast sandwich with coffee in the a.m., McDonald's and a Diet Coke for lunch, pizza and a beer for dinner, and *not* have problems getting pregnant?

Whom and What Do You Believe?

The commitment to assure yourself a healthy pregnancy and the optimum developmental environment for your baby needs to come from you. You need to do your homework—and not just on the latest gadgets to help a newborn sleep. Educate yourself about nutrition (as you are doing now by reading this book). Surround yourself with like-minded healthcare professionals to assist you, if necessary. What I mean by "like-minded" is partnering with a nurse, midwife, doctor, nutritionist, or other healthcare practitioner who understands the fundamental role nutrition plays in the human body and the special demands of conception and pregnancy. There are plenty of these practitioners who are specially trained to help you, but you may have to look outside "traditional" venues to find them.

It is a sad reality right now in the U.S. that many traditional medical doctors don't consider dietary causes or solutions when diagnosing and treating a patient.

When I discuss these topics with people, I often get questions that are dripping with resentment and frustration toward their "regular" doctor. "My doctor never told me to change my diet," or, "Why didn't she tell me that making dietary changes could make such a difference in restoring my health and my fertility?"

I understand their anger and resentment. I had the same reaction after spending nearly six years struggling with symptoms of MS only to learn I could have spared myself much of that horrific experience if I had stumbled upon the concept of nutrition as medicine much earlier. When I talked to my neurologist about the rumors I was hearing that dietary changes could help reverse symptoms, he told me, "You can try that if you want, but that's not going to help you." I remember that statement all too well. Here's a newsflash for you: it did help me. Throughout a three-year-long, intense nutritional overhaul, I slowly regained my mobility, stamina, and mental clarity. I got my life back. Food is powerful.

Our medical professionals who practice "traditional" medicine do so for the same reason I am writing this book: They want to resolve illness and help people live happy, productive lives. They go about their work, in most cases, with the highest degree of integrity, compassion, and dedication. But in many cases their training is old school.

They are trained to diagnose and treat conditions, diseases, and injuries with pharmaceutical drugs, high-tech diagnostic equipment, and other advanced technologies, many of which help save lives every day. The unfortunate development in our medical system is that our traditionally trained healthcare providers receive their education—and eventually their compensation—from a healthcare system that is largely directed and influenced by the pharmaceutical and insurance industries. I've had many medical doctors admit to me that the training they received on nutrition in medical school amounted to no more than two to four weeks at the most.

Unless they invest their own time and money on an educational path outside of medical school, they learn very little about the advances in nutrigenomics, epigenetics and nutritional sciences.

The reality is this: *Just because your doctor doesn't know about something doesn't mean it isn't true.*

Waking Up to the Positive Impact of Nutrition

Many of you have started to realize that nutrition has an enormous impact on your health status and ability to conceive, and that taking drugs alone isn't a "health strategy." These realizations may have you seeking a different philosophical approach to your fertility or future pregnancy, or how other health conditions are treated. New emphasis is being placed on therapies that use to be considered "alternative" by Americans, such as therapeutic massage, acupuncture, homeopathy, chiropractic, and yes, nutrition. In fact, in 2012 health-seekers in the U.S. spent a whopping 14.7 billion dollars out-of-pocket on non-traditional types of practitioners and an additional 12.8 billion dollars on natural product supplements.[23]

According to the Academy of Integrative Health Medicine, the big bucks being directed to non-traditional approaches in healthcare have caused an increase in research, which is validating the value these approaches offer.

The demands for alternative healthcare did not go unnoticed among traditional medical doctors either. Back in 1991, one doctor, Doctor Jeffrey Bland, saw the trends and recognized the benefits of integrating concepts of individual biochemistry with approaches to nutrition in an effort to create a personalized, systems-based approach to medicine. In the early years, Doctor Bland's ideas took the form of a research and training platform for healthcare practitioners who were interested in moving away from one-size-fits-all medicine. This new philosophical approach to medicine was termed "functional medicine." Since its inception, Doctor Bland's "functional medicine" exploded into a new paradigm for healthcare and is managed, worldwide, by the Institute for Functional Medicine (IFM).[24]

IFM's approach to healthcare has allowed a welcomed shift in medical practices to include a comprehensive approach that incorporates the mind, body, and spirit. Today, IFM administers an intensive, educational and certification program that is offered around the globe. They manage a database of thousands of providers in 92 countries worldwide that are certified in "functional medicine."[25]

According to the IFM organization, "functional medicine offers a therapeutic model for healthcare providers that addresses the underlying causes of disease, not just the symptoms." In the IFM model, "lifestyle, environmental and dietary factors lay the foundation for understanding the progression of disease and the function of the human body as a whole." It's an exciting new approach to medicine that undoubtedly will continue to grow rapidly around the globe.

You can learn more about The Institute for Functional Medicine by accessing its website at www.ifm.org. The web site includes a feature to search IFM's directory of certified healthcare providers by zip code and will list those in your area along with their specialty (internal medicine, gynecology, obstetrics, fertility, and so forth).

Strategic Pregnancy-Planning—Nutrition Matters

Let's make *your* health a priority. *Now* is the time to implement a strategy for a healthy pregnancy.

Optimal health is critical to ensuring your attempt at conception is successful, and once successful, that mother and baby have an optimal chance at wellness.

As hopeful new parents, the time for euphoria will come, but right now I want you to be strategic and focused, making short-term decisions for long-term benefit.

Your first job as loving, responsible future parents is to improve your overall health. Doing so will increase your fertility, increase your chances of a healthy pregnancy, and eventually reward you with your bundle of joy.

If you are six to twelve months away from your desired time frame for conception, please turn to Chapter 2 to get started.

CHAPTER 2

How to Find Fertility: Causes, Signs, Symptoms, and Tracking

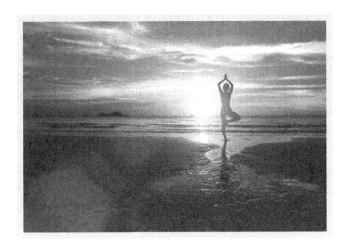

"Health is a state of complete harmony of the body, mind and spirit.

"When one is free from physical disabilities and mental distractions, the gates of the soul open."

—B.K.S. Iyengar

Understanding Unexplained Infertility

You may be one of the lucky couples who are able to conceive easily, seemingly if you just look at each other the right way. But that is not the good fortune most couples experience. In fact, it is more common for a woman *not* to get pregnant from her first attempt.

In the next couple of pages, I want to share with you some information and statistics about infertility in the hope of extinguishing any confusion, guilt, fear, or other bad feelings you're carrying around about this. *Infertility is not your fault or that of your partner.* Issues with fertility are no more your fault than having poor vision. Some people are genetically predisposed to specific health conditions. I am predisposed to having an autoimmune condition (MS). You might be predisposed to high blood pressure, migraine headaches, or infertility. None of us can control all the complex biochemical and metabolic processes going on inside our bodies. However, there are some areas we can control. The key is that we must know about them to effect change. Let me explain: It is good news for those dealing with infertility.

Research scientists are hot on the trail of two fascinating areas of study called nutrigenomics and epigenetics, which you read about in Chapter 1. What they are teaching us is that our genes respond to what we eat. If that didn't give you pause when you read it in the last chapter, take a second to think about it now. Changing what you eat doesn't just alter your weight or eliminate heartburn. It changes how your genetic code reacts during various stages of your life, and even in later generations.[1] You will start hearing more about both of these areas in upcoming years because both will continue to influence food manufacturing and governmental guidelines on nutrition. Eating healthy to minimize or resolve health issues will become the norm instead of being considered hokey-pokey nonsense. This is great news for me as a nutritionist because people will stop giving me that deer-in-the-headlights look when I tell them to stop overloading on carbs, soda, and sugary desserts.

The other encouraging trend here is that more and more people, like you, are not just sticking their heads in the sand, pretending that you are superhuman and don't have any genetic weaknesses or bad eating habits. You are educating yourself and dedicating the necessary time and effort into figuring out what steps you can take to overcome your inherited and biological weaknesses before they manifest.

As discussed in Chapter 1, pregnancy rates have fallen to a record low in the U.S. as of 2013, and cases of infertility are on the rise. In fact, infertility affects 8–12 percent of couples worldwide. 10.9 percent of women in the U.S. between the ages of fifteen and forty-four have impaired fertility.[2] These discouraging statistics do not include women dealing with secondary infertility—an inability to conceive their second child—which affects an additional three-plus million women, according to the National Center for Health Statistics.[3]

That is more than 7.5 million women. Of those, approximately 40–50 percent are due to infertility issues with the male, which includes issues with low sperm concentration, poor sperm motility (movement), and/or abnormal sperm development.[4]

The World Health Organization defines infertility this way:

Infertility is a disease of the reproductive system defined by failure to achieve the clinical pregnancy after 12 months or more of regular unprotected sexual intercourse.[5]

According to a study published in the Journal of Human Reproduction Science, 38 percent of women will get pregnant after one month, but the majority of women who were having sex each month during their peak time of fertility took three to six months to conceive. Hardly a "one and done" scenario for most women.

Do not be too quick to label yourself infertile, even if you're in your mid to late thirties and have been trying to get pregnant for over a year. The National Institute of Environmental Health Sciences conducted a study and found that the majority of women up to age thirty-nine (whose male partner was under the age of forty) who did not become pregnant in their first year of trying, did become pregnant in their second year—without any medical assistance.[6] Implementing a nutrition and lifestyle strategy will help decrease that time frame and increase your odds of success, despite age-related declining hormone levels.

Clearly—for most couples—getting pregnant takes planning, timing, and lots of patience. After reading this book, you will understand that your health strategy must include both the man and the woman; it will require you to take a close look at what you are putting into your body, and it will convince you to allow six to eight months *before* trying to conceive.

Is Your Current Diet Enhancing Fertility or Damaging It?

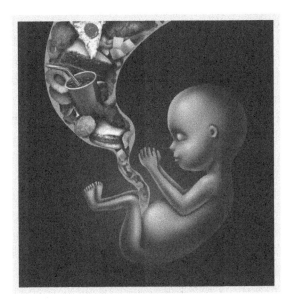

When we eat food, drink a beverage, inhale a scent, odor, or substance—or apply chemically laden lotions, creams, makeup, hair dyes, shampoos, conditioners, and more to our body—it all gets shuttled through the digestive system and eventually broken down into molecules. These molecules then get directed through various metabolic pathways that determine how the body will use them.

As a hopeful future parent, your goal is to deliver nourishing, beneficial, health-supportive molecules to your body's internal systems. You can accomplish this by paying close attention to what is in your diet and what types of things you need to avoid—exactly what we will cover throughout this book.

If your diet consists of too much junk, the molecules you will send coursing through your body will be toxic, creating havoc in cellular communication, poor absorption in the GI tract, dysfunction in your internal filtration and detoxification processes, impairment of the immune system, and a long list of other possible negative outcomes—all of which can contribute to infertility.

A fertility-boosting nutritional and lifestyle strategy is imperative for success if you are planning on having a baby. Still doubting? Here are a few additional key facts:

- Inflammation in the gut and elsewhere in the body can minimize nutrient absorption which can lead to deficiencies in available nutrients needed for healthy sperm, egg, and hormone production, which determines successful conception. (Gut health is so critical to fertility that I dedicated an entire chapter to it—Chapter 3.)[7] Exposure to toxic chemicals in foods, as well as heavy metals and radiation, can damage the DNA in our cells, which then affects gene expression that can negatively impact physiology and fertility health. Research has shown that long-term exposure to certain toxins—including pesticides, lead, cadmium, marijuana smoke, bisphenols found in plastic containers (which can leach into food and water), dry-cleaning chemicals, paint fumes, formaldehyde found in air fresheners, deodorants, and floor polish—damages human sperm development.[8]
- Consuming dairy products that are made from cows fed with hormone additives can disrupt the entire

endocrine system, leading to hormonal imbalances which can cause male infertility, as well as polycystic ovary syndrome and endometriosis in women.[9] After the age of thirty, your chances of conceiving in any given month diminish. Odds continue to decrease to the age of forty, after which they drop sharply. If you are in either of these age groups, adopting a healthy nutrition strategy will help bolster your hormone production and thereby improve your odds of conceiving.

Causes of Infertility in Women

There is a long list of health conditions, illnesses, and diseases that affect fertility and pregnancy. Immediately below are the ones you will read about most often: endometriosis, dysmenorrhea, and polycystic ovary syndrome (PCOS). A few other less common conditions are listed as well.

- Endometriosis—research is now considering whether this is an inflammatory condition with possible gut involvement. Studies show that 30–40 percent of women with endometriosis are infertile, and 6–15 percent of infertile women have endometriosis.[10]
- Dysmenorrhea or amenorrhea—secondary dysmenorrhea is excessive pain, cramping, and feeling of pressure in the abdomen during the menstrual cycle. It is connected to infertility when it evolves into other disorders involving the reproductive organs, such as endometriosis, uterine fibroids, or an infection. Secondary amenorrhea is often diagnosed in women who have their menstrual cycle stop after having a normal cycle. Both secondary dysmenor-

rhea and amenorrhea are connected to infertility and poor nutrition.[11]

- Polycystic Ovary Syndrome (PCOS)—PCOS is a common disorder of the endocrine system among women in their reproductive years. Women with PCOS usually will have at least two of the following conditions:

  1. Absence of ovulation, irregular periods, or no periods.
  2. High levels of androgen hormones indicated by excess body or facial hair.
  3. Cysts on one or both ovaries.

PCOS is strongly associated with insulin resistance, often caused by a diet high in carbohydrates and sugar.[12]

- Digestive issues—yeast overgrowth (Candida albicans), parasites, bacterial overgrowth, gut flora imbalance, and allergies. Gut disturbances are extremely common in the U.S. population today. The damage and inflammation they cause can be pervasive throughout the body.
- Bacterial vaginosis (BV)—the most common vaginal disorder in reproductive-age women. It is associated with infertility, pre-term births, endometriosis, pelvic inflammatory disease, and increased risk of HIV.

Health Conditions and Diseases That May Cause Female Infertility

- Obesity or being underweight
- Eating disorders

- Chronic stress
- Chlamydia
- Food allergies
- Poor liver detoxification
- Hashimoto or Graves' disease—Thyroiditis
- Insulin Resistance and blood sugar imbalance
- Mercury or other heavy metal poisoning
- Abnormal sperm production or function
- Abnormal delivery of sperm
- Overexposure to chemicals and toxins
- Damage related to cancer and cancer treatments
- Ovulation disorder
- Uterine or cervical abnormalities
- Fallopian tube damage or blockage
- Primary ovarian insufficiency (early menopause)
- Pelvic adhesions
- Delayed puberty
- Kidney disease or diabetes
- Amenorrhea (absence of menstruation)
- Celiac disease
- Cushing's disease

(Murray and Pizzorno, revised 2012)[13]

Causes of Infertility in Men

With over six million couples in the U.S. affected by infertility, half of them involve male infertility. Nearly 30 percent of these couples are impacted solely by male infertility.[14] Although it is most typical for the female to seek out infertility or medical assistance when pregnancy has not been achieved, it invariably leads to an analysis of the future dad's health in order to get a comprehensive view of all the issues with which a couple might be faced.

Most male infertility is due to abnormal sperm count or quality. Research has shown a strong connection between fertility and the number of sperm in an ejaculation. In 90 percent of the cases of low sperm count, the cause is abnormally low sperm production. (About two hundred million sperm will be present in an ejaculation, but only forty actually make it anywhere close to an egg—talk about swimming upstream without a paddle!)[15] *The Encyclopedia of Natural Medicine* gives a good list of typical causes of male infertility, along with causes of low sperm count.[16]

Health Conditions and Disease That May Cause Male Infertility

- Deficient sperm production
- Duct obstruction
- Congenital defects
- Post-infectious obstruction
- Cystic fibrosis
- Vasectomy
- Ejaculatory dysfunction
- Premature ejaculation
- Retrograde ejaculation
- Disorders of accessory glands
- Infection
- Inflammation
- Antisperm antibodies
- Coital disorders (anxiety before or after sex)
- Defects in sexual performance

- Premature withdrawal
- Erectile dysfunction

(Murray and Pizzorno, revised 2012)[17]

Possible Causes of Low Sperm Count

- Increased scrotal temperature
- Tight-fitting clothing
- Varicose veins around the testes
- Environment (smoking, excessive alcohol use, recreational drug use
- Obesity
- Exposure to pollution
- Heavy metals (lead, mercury, and so forth)
- Organic solvents
- Pesticides
- Diet
- High intake of saturated fats
- Deficient intake of fruits, vegetables and whole grains
- Reduced intake of dietary fiber
- Excess exposure to synthetic estrogen

(Murray and Pizzorno, revised 2012)[18]

The first step in improving sperm count, quality, and motility is to control the external factors that can cause damage or impairment. These factors include:

- Control the temperature of the scrotal sac by wearing appropriate (loose) clothing and underwear, periodically taking a cold shower, or even applying ice to the scrotum. Elevated scrotal temperature is a common cause of infertility in men.

- Eliminate any existing infections such as urinary tract, prostate, or those from sexually transmitted diseases.
- Reduce or eliminate exposure to environmental toxins such as heavy metals, radiation, pollution, and so forth.
- Eliminate cigarette smoking, excessive alcohol consumption and recreational drug use.
- Reduce excess weight.
- Follow a nutritious, optimal, whole-foods diet plan. Avoid, sugar, gluten, toxins in food sources.

(Murray and Pizzorno, revised 2012)[19]

Except for scrotal temperature cooling, all the above issues are addressed in the Conception Strategy for Men that follows later in this chapter.

A quick story about the power of food. A female client of mine in her mid-thirties came to me for nutrition counseling relating to MS symptoms. As I reviewed her client intake form, it was immediately apparent that her health status was complicated by other factors. Her thyroid had been removed several years earlier for a benign thyroid nodule, she was obese, borderline pre-diabetic, was under a lot of stress, and had amenorrhea—hadn't had a menstrual cycle for many months. Within three to four months on a healthy dietary program, not only was the weight coming off fairly rapidly, but her monthly periods returned and hormone activity was restored. Changing the food molecules that she put in her body fostered a change in cell communication, improved nutrient absorption, balanced blood sugar levels, and got those hormones sending proper signals once again.

Hopefully you're getting the picture—you *are* what you eat—literally.

Diagnostic Testing and Tracking Signs of Fertility

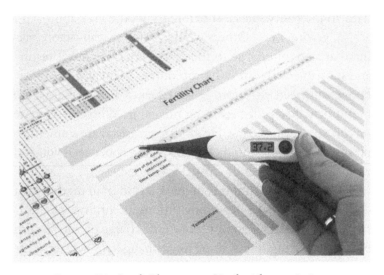

Source: Big Stock Photo.com. Used with permission.

Some of you may have concerns about infertility, and although you haven't yet sought advice from a fertility expert, you're considering it.

Most medical doctors who specialize in infertility have a great deal of expertise in this area. They will leave few stones unturned and will dig deep into your medical and gynecological history to look for clues as to what may be causing infertility. A physical exam will be conducted, along with blood tests to check levels of female hormones, thyroid hormones, prolactin, male hormones, and signs of other contributing health conditions or diseases such as HIV, hepatitis, chlamydia, or other infections.

There are also other tests they may perform if they suspect something physiological, such as a fallopian-tube blockage, a uterine defect or obstruction, or to determine if the follicles in the ovaries are working normally.

Some of you may elect to move right to full-blown testing with an infertility specialist before trying the DIY approach I am suggesting here. Others would prefer to wait before taking that step, often due to the costs of out-of-pocket testing and subsequent IUI or IVF procedures. Many of you already know you need to improve your health before taking the monumental step of becoming pregnant. Wherever you are on this spectrum is okay. Healthcare decisions are immensely personal ones and should be made privately between you and your significant other or trusted loved one.

What I want to impress upon you is that no matter what decisions you make regarding infertility testing or treatments, it is always a good idea to take charge of your health by implementing sound nutritional changes. Whatever route you take to achieving conception, creating a healthy environment for your fetus and maintaining your own health during pregnancy are critical to delivering a healthy baby.

Self-Testing for Fertility and Ovulation

In a woman, there are a few telltale signs of fertility that you can monitor yourself. If you don't mind putting in the effort, doing so may result in determining the time of month when you are fertile. Armed with that information, you will then have a window of opportunity to engage in sexual intercourse and have a higher probability of conceiving.

Technology advances have permeated women's health issues at almost the same pace as entertainment, news, and online shopping. There are a many apps available for fertility tracking, some providing basic basal temperature tracking, and others that allow the user to monitor habits, cravings, emotions and cramp pain levels from month to month. Some have a cost or membership fee; others don't. Some have a tracking mechanism only for a woman's fertility cycle; a couple offer tracking for a woman and a man.

Read through the different self-test methods below, pick one (or more) that makes sense for your schedule and budget, do your own investigative work, and then get yourself organized and let the tracking begin! For those of you who prefer an old-fashioned method of tracking, a few traditional methods are mentioned in the section that follows.

Whether or not you decide to track your fertility, or irrespective of the method you choose, be aware that no method is foolproof. Fertility apps and websites that rely on accurate data entry and estimates cannot be relied upon to accurately predict a fertility "window."

I should mention that I have no ties whatsoever to any of these companies or their products. I also have not received any compensation for mentioning any of them here. Having said all that, I do have a favorite that I identified, which is the Conceivable product. I am impressed by this product's unique focus on identifying the most fertile time for a woman, and the customized nutrition recommendations offered to increase fertility. It is not the cheapest product on the market, but might offer the most value and reportedly high accuracy.

Ultimately, you need to do your own homework and find the one best suited for your lifestyle and goals.

Tech-Savvy Methods of Tracking Fertility

Where there's a problem to solve, there's an app to solve it for you...or in this case, track it for you, and there are a lot of them available to choose from. I highlighted just a few. Those with an asterisk were rated by *Healthline* online magazine as "The Best Fertility Apps of 2017"[20] (not listed in order of Healthline rating).

Conceivable*—www.conceivable.com. Based on principles of Chinese medicine and acupuncture, this product provides everything under the sun to help its users get pregnant. Its founder was a fertility acupuncturist. *Conceivable* will drop-ship supplements, provide meal plans, and advise on nearly every part of health that could impact pregnancy, based on ongoing cycle information.

Cost: Download is free, ninety-nine dollars monthly subscription inclusive of supplements and personalized services.

Kindara*—www.kindara.com. Monitors basal body temperature and cervical fluid to learn about hormone levels in your body and tell you the best time to conceive. Works alongside an oral thermometer called "Wink," which retails for 129 dollars and syncs automatically to the app.

Cost: Free, "Wink" thermometer, 129 dollars.

Glow*—www.glowing.com. Pinpoints a woman's fertility cycle using personalized data to help her conceive faster.

Cost: Free with the option of contributing to a mutual assistance program which can be used towards fertility treatments if Glow doesn't help you conceive in ten months. Cost: Free on iOS and Android.

Natural Cycles*—www.naturalcycles.com. This app can determine the best times for trying to get pregnant using your mobile device, a thermometer, and optional ovulation test strips to measure LH hormone the day before ovulation.

Will signal with a red or a green day—green means you can't get pregnant; red means you can get pregnant.

Cost: Download free on iOS and Android, annual subscription fee of 69.90 dollars which includes a basal thermometer.

Fitbit/Ava—www.avawomen.com. The Ava is an armband similar to the fitness and activity bands that are so popular. It is worn only during sleep and tracks nine different physical indicators, which change during windows of fertility. Ava claims to be one of few fertility trackers that will tell you in real time when you're most fertile. Manufacturer says their product is especially useful for women of "advanced maternal age" (over thirty-five years old).

Cost: 199 dollars

There are many others besides those highlighted above; in fact, there are literally hundreds of products. Here are a few others you might include in your product search: Ovia,* Yono, Clue,* TempDrop, Dot,* Fertility Friend,* Welltwigs, ClearPlan. Clearblue, My Pregnancy Today, Pink Pad, BabyBump, and I'm Expecting.

*Rated by *Healthline* online magazine as "The Best Fertility Apps of 2017"

Traditional Fertility-Tracking Methods

If you prefer a more traditional, low-cost, "old-school" method of tracking your fertility, below are a few methods you might consider.

1. Monitor Cervical Fluid

   During the first part of the reproductive cycle, a high concentration of estrogen causes the uterus and cervix to secrete a watery fluid that supports sperm transport and survival. This watery fluid is clear—

some would describe it as "slippery" in the beginning of ovulation—and changes to a sticky and creamy consistency as you continue through ovulation. All women will have this production of fluid in varying quantity and duration. You can pinpoint your most fertile time of the month by becoming familiar with the production of this fluid. For most women, your most fertile time period is when the cervical fluid is produced in the largest quantity. Some women will have this for a day, while others will have up to two weeks of cervical fluid.

2. Monitor Cervical Opening

During ovulation, your cervix is open to its widest point; it closes after ovulation is complete. Depending on an individual woman's anatomy, it is possible for some women to feel the opening of the cervix with a finger. By checking it on a regular basis, you will start to notice the changes in the opening, giving you signs of when ovulation is occurring.

3. Track Basal Body Temperature

Tracking basal body temperature is the more common, self-administered approach to tracking your fertility. Here's how it's done:

- Purchase a basal body temperature thermometer from your local drug store.
- Take your temperature as close to the same time every morning as possible, preferably before you are too active.
- Take your temperature either vaginally or under your arm. Whichever method you choose you should remain consistent with it each time you check going forward.

- Once the thermometer beeps, record the temperature reading on a piece of paper with the date and time.

When you are ovulating, your temperature should be between 97 and 98.2 degrees Fahrenheit, and at least 0.3 degrees above that after ovulation. Your temperature will drop back to pre-ovulation levels right before you menstruate.

You should be aware that a condition exists in a very small number of women that will cause an irregular fluctuation in body temperature even though ovulation (egg release) is not occurring. It is called "anovulatory cycle." Your doctor can run tests to determine if you have this condition. The upside is that hormone balance can often be achieved and normal ovulation cycles restored by changing what you eat, so keep reading!

Some women will chart a constant temperature every day with no fluctuations whatsoever, no matter what time they wake up or what the air temperature is. The longer you track, the more you will understand how your body works and its patterns relating to fertility.

Other Signs of Ovulation and Fertility

As part of your tracking, pay attention to other clues that your body may be giving you. Some of the most common are listed below. By recording how you feel over a period of two, three, or four months, you may discover other patterns and signals indicating that your fertility is peaking and ovulation is about to occur. Many of the apps listed in the previous section will allow you to enter some of this information in the app and then use it in their tracking algorithm.

- Increased libido
- Sensations in the area of the ovaries
- Mood changes, "down-in-the-dumps" feeling
- Changes in appetite
- Period "irregularities such as irregular cycle, heavy bleeding, cramping, clotting, short cycle, or PMS.

The next chapter is about a topic that most people will be inclined to skip over, but please don't. The information it contains might very well be the most critical to your understanding of why nutrition matters in supporting your health as a future mommy or daddy. Before you take a sneak peek at what this mysterious, upcoming chapter is about, make a pact with me right now that you will read it and digest as much of it as you can (no pun intended). Your body, and that of the little one you will create, is more of a miracle than you could ever imagine. The next chapter reveals one of the most spectacular, magical parts of the human body, and the critical role it plays in your fertility.

CHAPTER 3

You and Your Baby Are Bugged: Your Microbiome and How It Affects Fertility

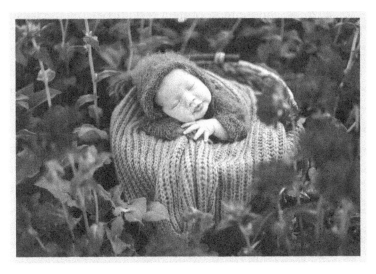

Source: BigStockPhoto.com. Used with permission.

"Miracles, in the sense of phenomena we cannot explain, surround us on every hand: life itself is the miracle of miracles."

—*George Bernard Shaw*

For those of you who followed my advice at the end of Chapter 2 and made the mental commitment to stick with me through this next chapter, you deserve a pat on the back. This is one of those chapters where a lot of people will say, "Aw shucks. I don't really need to read *this*." But, in fact, you do, or at least I hope you do. I'll explain why shortly, but before I do I would like to try to make you more comfortable with a typically uncomfortable topic.

You know those conversations you've had with people where you try to explain to yourselves why in the world a doctor would choose to become a certain type of specialist? There's no scientific basis for the opinions expressed. It's all based on the "ick" factor, with gynecology and gastroenterology (the GI system or "gut") usually eliciting the most ardent protest with a loud "eeewwww!" Seriously, who in their right mind wants to spend their career examining a woman's female parts inside and out? Or how about those medical students who decide to focus on the organs that produce human excrement...i.e., poop? To quote Doctor Gershon from his book *The Second Brain,* "No poet would ever write an ode to the intestine."[1] It's just not easy to romanticize the colon.

We all know the human body is indeed miraculous in how it functions. It is challenging to argue the point that the mysteries of the universe may lay within our ability to procreate, which makes gynecology and obstetrics very intriguing, to say the least. But in my opinion, and that of more recent scientific research, one of the most fascinating areas of the human body is the human microbiome, the largest part of which is located in the gastrointestinal system.

The gut microbiome, and its connection to other areas in the human body, is where the medical and biochemical magic is really happening, and there's plenty of cutting-edge science to back me up. Furthermore, its effect on your fertility, vaginal microbiome, fetus, and eventually your newborn is nothing short of riveting.

What Is the Human Microbiome?

The human body contains an ecosystem—a community of living organisms that interact with each other and with the non-living things in their environment. These organisms are also called "microbes" and together they form various communities made up of bacteria, viruses, fungi, and other substances; collectively they are called the human microbiome.[2] (For purposes of consistency and simplicity, I will occasionally use the terms "bacteria" and "microbes" interchangeably. Bacteria are a type of microbe and one of the most common, but other types of organisms are considered microbes as well.)

Bacteria are part of every life-form on our planet. Indeed, bacteria have been around for over 3.5 billion years and have been a fundamental part of the creation of new life-forms.[3] Throughout our evolutionary process as humans, mankind has merged with bacteria. In fact, we became so intertwined with bacteria that, in our present-day form, bacteria is part of every cell in our body.

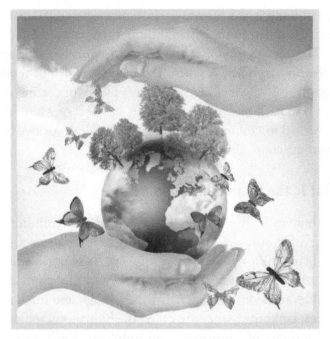

Source: AdobeStock.com. Used with permission.

Beyond this interconnectedness exists an interdependency as well. Humans need bacteria to remain healthy and some types of bacteria and microbes need the environment provided by the human body to survive.[4] In *Your Baby's Microbiome* (Harmon & Wakeford, 2017), it is described this way:

In effect, the human body is a complex ecosystem made up of human cells and microorganisms existing together. So you could say we are all part human, part microbe.[5]

Normal, beneficial bacteria take up residence in the human body in the gut and other areas during the birth process and remain there throughout an individual's lifetime.[6] Current research is still trying to determine just how many microbes reside on and in the typical human body as compared to human cells. Even though we don't have an exact number, estimates are that it may be as high as one hundred to one—*one hundred times more microbes than human cells.* There are literally thousands of different species of bacteria that live on and inside a human body, and they all carry an incredible amount of genetic material.[7] Researchers from the Human Microbiome Project estimate that there is "several hundred times more genetic material within our microbes than there is carried within our human genes."[8]

Where Are the Bacteria?

Bacteria in and on the human body are so prolific it's almost easier to tell you where you won't find them. Research continues as to whether or not bacteria are present in the blood, heart, liver, pancreas, and ovaries. But there is definitive science that shows commensal bacteria—that is, beneficial bacteria—are present in every part of the human body that has exposure to the outside world.

One obvious area is the skin, which is highly absorbent. I sat in on a lecture given by Doctor Keesha Ewers in April 2017, during which she described our skin as a functioning, highly absorbable organ and anything it comes in contact with—such as lotions, creams, insect repellant, sunscreen, makeup, hair dyes, and so forth—is assimilated so effectively it is no different than if we were *eating* those things.[9] Suddenly I found myself rethinking all the products I use on my face, skin, nails and scalp. Do you sit down at your dinner table and scoop out a couple tablespoons of sun screen or hair dye and toss it in with your salad? Probably not. But thinking about how absorbent our skin is, is definitely worthy of more respect and consideration when choosing skin and hair care products.

Other areas where our helpful microscopic friends can be found include the eyes, ears, and nose—all are openings where bacteria can gain entry to the body. And then there is your respiratory system. Based on a rate of twelve breaths per minute, and depending on the time of year, the average person could inhale up to 36,000 bacteria every hour, making our lungs, mouth, throat, and airway passages prime hosts for bacteria, good and not-so-good.[10]

Other not-so-obvious examples of where these co-inhabitants are found include the brain and urinary tract, as well as the urine itself (even low levels are found in a healthy individual).

The brain is particularly interesting because it was always thought to be a sterile environment, but neuroscientists are diligently researching its close connection with the gut, and the bidirectional relationship that exists between the gut bacteria and the brain.[11]

(Now, in case some of you are starting to rethink that commitment I asked you to make at the beginning to stay with me through this entire chapter, don't bail out on me now. This is the point when it starts to get really interesting, and I promise you will start to understand the relevance to your future son or daughter.)

Researchers refer to this bidirectional relationship as the "gut–brain axis" and it is considered one of the new frontiers of neuroscience.[12] What we're learning from this cutting-edge research is that the healthy development of a newborn's gut microbiome is critical to the development of the central nervous system and mental health.[13] Disruption of these developmental patterns during early infancy (first three years of life) can potentially lead to mental health problems later in life, such as depression, anxiety, or cognitive issues.[14]

The Role Microbes Play in the Human Body and How to Protect Them

Sometimes microbes contribute to sickness, but in most cases they live in harmony within the body where they have taken up residence. The potentially harmful microbes—the bad guys—only become a risk to our health when they start to outnumber the good guys, and there are a number of factors that can cause that to happen. Not only are most microbes friendly to their human host—they provide important functions critical to our survival, and in some cases help prevent certain disease conditions[15].

We can trace research on the human microbiome back to the early 1600s, around the time the microscope was invented, but advances in genomics, epigenetics and other similar areas of scientific study have currently caused a ground-swell of interest within the scientific community. The Human Microbiome Project, (HMP) began in 2008 with the mission to research and examine the role microbes play in human health and disease.[16] What we're learning from their research will continue to influence changes in modern medicine, how we fight disease, our nutrition standards, and food manufacturing, to name a few. Eventually, our knowledge about the microbiome and how a newborn is "seeded" may result in modifications to our birthing processes as well.

Although scientists are just beginning to scratch the surface of the roles microbes play in our existence as human beings, we do know their health-promoting functions in a few key areas. To stay focused on the topics of fertility, conception, and pregnancy, except for the areas that are relevant, I have chosen not to go into detail on most of these despite how significant and fascinating each one is to our well-being.

Some of the key areas influenced by our internal microbiome environment include:

- Genetic expression—the gut microbiome communicates with human cells to switch genes on and off, which is the main "switch" for the body's ability to express a state of good health or a disease state.[17] Knowing this gives new emphasis to the phrase "gut feeling"!

- Immune system—the gut contains the largest part of your immune system and actually controls certain types of immune cells.[18] Through the interaction of these two systems, the immune system responds to inflammatory responses that begin in the gut and then travel to the brain, ultimately sending signals to the rest of your body.[19]

- Body weight and composition—resident microbes have a major impact on digestion by breaking down proteins, lipids, and carbohydrates, in essence serving as the gatekeeper as to whether we are thin or obese.[20]

- Mental health—the gut microbiome is vital to brain development and has been linked to behavior, anxiety, stress, and stress-related diseases. There is also a direct link between the gut bacteria and the nervous system.[21]

- Gut function—commensal microbes have a significant role in the digestion process and absorption of nutrients. From within their home in the GI tract, they produce compounds like vitamins and anti-inflammatories that our genes can't.[22]

As scientists expand their research on the human microbiome, they continue to learn more about the areas within the human body that are impacted, if not controlled to varying degrees, by our bug population. They are also learning ways in which the bugs can be influenced, and one of the major ways is through diet and reducing exposure of the body to toxins. Below is a chart that outlines an excellent list of dos and don'ts for your microbiome.

Suggestions for Protecting Your Microbiome[23]

Do:	Avoid:
Eat plenty of fermented foods. Healthy choices include lassi, fermented grass-fed organic milk such as kefir, and fermented vegetables. Be sure you're getting enough vitamin K2, particularly important if you're taking a vitamin D3 supplement.	Antibiotics, unless absolutely necessary, especially during pregnancy and only on the advice of your physician. If you do take them, make sure to reseed your gut with fermented foods and/or a probiotic supplement.
Take a probiotic supplement. Probiotic supplements are on the list for pre-conception and pregnancy, but are especially important if your diet is low in fermented foods.	Conventionally-raised meats and other animal products are routinely fed low-dose antibiotics, plus genetically engineered grains loaded with glyphosate, which is widely known to kill many bacteria.

| Boost your soluble and insoluble fiber intake, focusing on vegetables, nuts, and seeds, including sprouted seeds. | Chlorinated and/or fluoridated water. Avoid excessive bathing/showers, which can kill more bacteria than drinking water. Avoid frequent visits to your local pool during pre-conception and pregnancy to avoid chlorine. |
| Get your hands dirty in the garden. Germ-free living may not be in your best interest, as the loss of healthy bacteria can have wide-ranging influence on your mental, emotional, and physical health. Exposure to bacteria and viruses can serve as "natural vaccines" that strengthen your immune system and provide long-lasting immunity against disease. Getting your hands dirty in the garden can help reacquaint your immune system with beneficial microorganisms on the plants and in the soil. | Processed foods. Excessive sugars, along with otherwise "dead" nutrients, feed pathogenic bacteria. Food emulsifiers such as polysorbate 80, carrageenan, and polyglycerols also appear to have an adverse effect on your gut flora. Unless 100 percent organic, they may also contain GMOs that tend to be heavily contaminated with pesticides such as glyphosate. |

Open your windows. For the vast majority of human history, the outside was always part of the inside, and at no moment during our day were we ever really separated from nature. Today, we spend 90 percent of our lives indoors. Research shows that opening a window and increasing natural airflow can improve the diversity and health of the microbes in your home, which in turn benefits you.	Agricultural chemicals, glyphosate (Roundup) in particular, is a known antibiotic and will actively kill many of your beneficial gut microbes if you eat foods contaminated with Roundup. This is especially true for wheat (bread).
Wash your dishes by hand instead of in the dishwasher. Recent research has shown that washing your dishes by hand leaves more bacteria on the dishes than dishwashers do, and that eating off these less-than-sterile dishes may actually decrease your risk of allergies by stimulating your immune system.	Antibacterial soap kills off both good and bad bacteria and contributes to the development of antibiotic resistance.

Source: Mercola, J., MD (2015). *"Research Reveals the Importance of Your Microbiome for Optimal Health"* Chart printed with modifications by Barbara Rodgers.

Why You Need to Be Bugged to
Have a Healthy Pregnancy

A lot of our discussion so far on the "microbiome" has been centered on the gut. Microscopically speaking, the bug environment in the gut looks very different than the friendly inhabitants that are found in the reproductive tissues. The important fact for you to know, however, is that the reproductive organs are tightly linked and regulated by the functions of the bacterial population found within the GI tract.[24] Scientists have known for a long time that the bacterial species found in the GI tract create and use enzymes that are required for processing and circulating estrogen.[25] Furthermore, if this bacterial group (known as the estrabolome), becomes altered, changes can occur in the circulating estrogen levels, which affect various reproductive functions, including pregnancy and fertility.[26] To say this a different way, if your gut microbiome is out of whack (as evidenced by ongoing digestive issues, chronic infections, a chronic disease, or an ongoing state of overall poor health), it can affect the health of your reproductive functions.

And the power of the bugs is not unique to women either. A male partner is at risk for an imbalance in the gut microbiome and infertility if dealing with conditions such as Crohn's disease, irritable bowel syndrome, ulcerative colitis, any active inflammation, poor nutrition, excessive alcohol use, smoking, recent surgical procedure, or ongoing use of many classes of medications.[27]

Hopefully, you're getting the picture that the human microbiome affects all aspects of reproduction, from the development of a cell into one that can be fertilized, fertilization, embryo migration, implantation, implications in early miscarriage, involvement in late pregnancy loss, poor health during gestation, infections during the birthing process, and preterm birth.[28]

In short, never underestimate the power of your guts' bugs!

Mom's Bugs, Pregnancy, and Baby

I saved some of the most sensational details (in my opinion) for last. Until very recently, most people believed that a woman's body provided an almost sterile environment for the growth and development of her baby. I should add that you weren't alone in your thinking. In fact, the womb being a sterile environment was a long-held belief among scientists as well. As I said, it is only with recent research that we have discovered that babies are being exposed to bacteria prior to being born. Don't let this news shatter your dreams of the beautiful, perfect miracle that is waiting for you on your delivery day. Your baby being "bugged" is a good thing. In studies, scientists have discovered small amounts of bacteria present in the womb, the placenta, and amniotic fluid.[29] They have even found bacteria in the fetus's intestines, which means your baby's microbiome becomes established much earlier than we thought, prior to birth.[30]

Science has yet to tell us definitively where these bacteria come from, but one theory is that they travel from the mother's oral microbiome (her mouth), through the blood stream and reach the fetus through the placenta, or some microbes might come from the mother's vagina and travel to the uterus.[31] There are several important takeaways from this data. First, it means that Mom's health and whether her gut bacteria is balanced and healthy matters a great deal in the healthy development and growth of her baby, including what types of diseases her child might be susceptible to later in life. It also points to the fact that, at least for some infants, the gut microbiome begins in utero and can be influenced by the health (including oral health) and diet of the mother during pregnancy.[32]

Childbirth and Seeding Your Baby's Microbiome

On the day of your "main event," your delivery day, a lot is happening, particularly in the baby's gut and microbiome. The way in which a baby enters this world—a vaginal birth or Caesarean—dramatically influences the diversity and composition of the baby's bacterial population, and by extension, the child's health for his or her entire life.[33] Remember: The bacteria we're talking about here are the "good guys."

In Toni Harman and Alex Wakeford's book, *Your Baby's Microbiome*, they describe the foundational process of "seeding" a newborn's microbiome beautifully and with clarity:

"The moment that the waters break (if they do) is the critical moment for the main seeding of the baby's microbiome. As soon as the membranes of the amniotic sac rupture, the baby is suddenly exposed to an influx of bacteria. In the birth canal, without the protection of the amniotic sac, the baby becomes coated in the mother's vaginal microbes, which the newborn skin soaks up like a sponge. The microbes enter the baby's eyes, ears, and nose, and make their way into the baby's mouth. The baby is covered with the bacteria; is swallowing the bacteria. That's the baby's first introduction to the world of bacteria, the world we all live in. That's the founding microbiome for that baby."[34]

These initial microbe settlers in your baby perform critical functions: They populate the baby's gut microbiome; help digest lactose during breastfeeding, which produces energy;

and they play a vital role in training the immune system to protect the baby from harmful bacteria and pathogens.

Babies born by Cesarean section will not have the exchange of fluids and vaginal material to populate the microbiome in the way a vaginal birth will. Without passing through the birth canal, the baby simply does not have the opportunity for exposure to the mother's microbes. In the case of a Csection, a doctor splits open the amniotic sac, at which point the baby will receive a flood of microbes that will enter its eyes, nose, ears and cover its skin, but those microbes will come from the air in the environment rather than from the birth canal.[35]

It is a different scenario if the Cesarean section is an emergency. In many cases where the Csection is not planned in advance, the baby is not removed until it is already in the birth canal, and perhaps even after the mother's waters have broken. These events provide the baby with exposure to the mother's vaginal microbes, even if for a shorter time.

There are many other aspects and considerations of proper seeding of your baby's microbiome that are, unfortunately, too detailed to get into for this book. For instance, there is the effect of a newborn being exposed to harmful bacteria or antibiotics shortly before or after delivery. Fascinating research is also underway to determine the impact of an en-caul birth (sac is intact) on the microbiome, as well as the effects of skin-to-skin contact or "swab-seeding" following a Cesarean section.

For anyone who is interested in learning more about these topics or the process and importance of newborn seeding I strongly encourage you to read *Your Baby's Microbiome* by Harmon and Wakeford (2016, Chelsea Green Publishing). It is an intricate, wonderfully written book based on the most current research on this mind-blowing area of medical research.

Your Microbiome and Breastfeeding

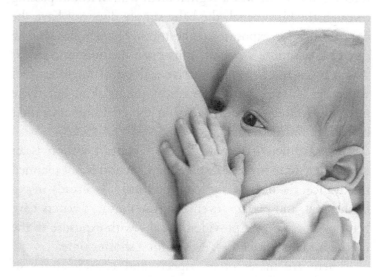

Source: StockAdobe.com. Used with permission.

It is fairly common knowledge that breastfeeding introduces the nutrients and microbial organisms to your newborn infant that stimulate the development of its immune system. What is not typically known is that it also supports proper development of major metabolic functions later in life, reduces the risk of premature babies developing retinopathy or other eye diseases later in life, decreases the risk of obesity, diabetes and intestinal diseases, and reduces the risk of heart disease in mothers who breastfeed for ten months or longer.[36] It is an essential role for a new mom that provides optimal nutrition to her newborn.

Earlier in this chapter, we described the importance of the seeding process of a newborn's microbiome. As babies pass through the birth canal (in a vaginal delivery), they are first exposed to the mother's vaginal bacteria before entering our environment. In many deliveries, a mom is given the opportunity for skin-to-skin contact of their newborn, which allows for the transfer of more bacteria from the mother's skin to the baby's skin.[37] Either immediately following delivery or sometime soon after, the newborn is allowed to breastfeed. With the baby's mouth well-seeded with lactobacilli bacteria from the birthing process, its digestive system is already equipped to break down the lactose in the milk, which helps to produce energy for the baby.

The breast fluid available to the infant for the first three to four days is not actually milk. It is colostrum, and happens to contain the exact nutrients needed in the first few hours and days of life to nourish the baby and provide the much-needed microbes for the gut. Colostrum is a watery substance with a sticky consistency. It is dense in nutrients—low in fat, high in protein, and loaded with antigens, antibodies, anti-inflammatories, and cells to stimulate growth.[38]

When mom's breast milk "comes in" (again, varies from woman-to-woman, but around three to four days following delivery), it also is rich in nutrients—vitamins, minerals, fats, carbohydrates (mostly in the form of lactose for energy), amino acids, and proteins. It also contains probiotics that feed good bacteria in the gut and support growth of additional gut bacteria.[39]

The wonder of a woman's body doesn't end with producing breast milk shortly after giving birth. As her baby grows, the nutrient values of her breast milk and the microbial content grow and evolve as well.[40] Research has shown that specific types of bacteria that were present in colostrum have changed considerably in the breast milk a month later. It is believed that this evolution of bacteria and nutrient content of breast milk accommodates the ongoing development of the infant immune system and neurological functions.[41]

This amazing process ensures that your baby receives the perfect recipe of nutrients through the many stages of development, including the development of a strong, healthy immune system and a properly seeded gut microbiome. If properly nurtured and nourished, both will continue to do their jobs for a lifetime.

Eating the Baby-Maker Way: What to Eat to Have a Healthy Pregnancy

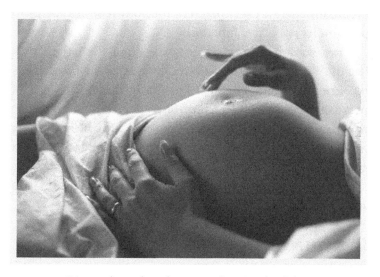

"A mother's joy begins when new life is stirring inside...

When a tiny heartbeat is heard for the very first time,

and a playful kick reminds her that she is never alone."

—*unknown author*

A Healthy Pregnancy Introduction

We nourish the body so all of its internal and external systems can perform the various functions necessary every second of every day for us to continue breathing, thinking, moving, talking, and so forth. In short, food becomes molecules and eventually energy. Every organ of the body requires energy to perform its respective function.

You will often hear women talk about the fatigue they feel during pregnancy, most typically during the first trimester. Energy is especially depleted during the early stages of pregnancy because of the added physiological changes occurring to support the pregnancy. You see a little belly forming in your mid-section, but there is a whole lot more than that going on. The list below will give you a small glimpse of the types of biological magic that occurs in the woman's body to support her pregnancy.[1]

Cardiovascular System

- Heart enlarges slightly.
- Heart rate and cardiac output increases.

- Blood pressure decreases during first half of pregnancy and returns to non-pregnant levels during second half.
- Plasma volume and red blood cell volume increases.
- Respiratory rate and oxygen consumption increases.

Gastrointestinal Tract, Food Intake, and Digestion

- Appetite increases.
- Senses of taste and smell are altered.
- Thirst increases.
- Gastrointestinal movement decreases.
- Efficiency of nutrient absorption increases.
- Gastroesophageal reflux becomes more common (increase in stomach acid).

Renal System

- Kidney filtration rate increases.
- Sodium retention increases.
- Total body water increases.

Energy Metabolism and Energy Balance

- Basal metabolic rate (BMR) increases.
- Body temperature increases.
- Fat mass, lean mass, and body weight increases.

There are incredibly complex changes going on in the female body, and the above list doesn't even include what is happening to support formation of the placenta or fetal development. Imagine the energy demands being placed on the various systems to make sure all of this happens. Your body is suddenly gearing up for a marathon without the weeks or months of training to prepare for it—of course you're tired!

"My Pregnancy Plate"

Supporting Mom's health with organic, nourishing whole foods is fundamental to sustaining the intense work her body needs to perform while carrying her baby. Hopefully, you're beginning to understand that this is no small task!

A mother's energy requirement increases by about 50 percent during pregnancy) because she is sharing her body's energy supply with her developing baby.[2] All nutrients consumed by the mother are used *first* by the baby and the balance is used by the mother. Pregnant mothers are truly "eating for two"!

It takes an average of 60,000 calories to make a baby over the nine-month gestation period, or an extra 300 to 400 calories per day.[3] Therefore, an average woman needs 2400 to 2600 calories a day when pregnant—less in the first trimester, more in the last trimester.[4] Remember: Calories are a method to measure energy, and food equals energy.

It is monumentally important to supplement your energy reserves by eating high-calorie, healthy, organic foods, as well as staying away from things that are not supportive such as foods that are full of chemicals or toxins. Lifestyle issues that have a detrimental effect on overall health should also be eliminated—particularly smoking and drinking alcohol.

Recent research is showing that babies born to women who gain the *healthiest* weight during pregnancy—not weight gain from milkshakes, cookies and chips!—were at the *least* risk of developing problems, both before birth and after.[5]

A diet high in proteins is important, especially complete proteins. Complete proteins come from animal sources and contain all the amino acids required for all your bodily functions. They are the building blocks of all bodily tissues and cells, and they are essential for hormone and antibody production during pregnancy.

During pregnancy (and after delivery if nursing) a diet should consist of sprouted nuts and seeds, non-starchy organic vegetables, a small number of legumes and beans, fresh organic fruits, pure unrefined oils, wild-caught fish, grass-fed antibiotic-free and hormone-free meat and poultry, organic eggs, and organic unsweetened nut milks. For a condensed, graphical depiction of what a healthy diet looks like during pregnancy, please take a look at "My Holistic Pregnancy Plate" on the next page. I created this graphic so you can visualize in totality what your daily food intake should look like.

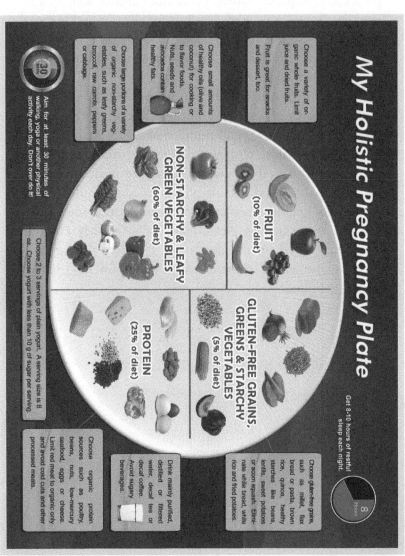

Image created by Marty Laudato, Marina Graphics, LLC

Food Nuances

Depending on the food category, there are nuances with particular foods that make them good choices during pregnancy or not, depending on your biochemical makeup and overall health. The risk of developing various health conditions or complications during pregnancy can be dramatically reduced by paying close attention to what you eat and don't eat, which means it is well worth your time to know a little more about some of your favorite foods and the role they will play in your overall diet.

Take potatoes, for instance. Most people love potatoes, I happen to be one of them. In my past, you would never find me turning down an order of French fries or a baked potato loaded with butter, bacon and chives. Potatoes contain a concentrated source of some great nutrients like vitamin B6, C, dietary fiber, potassium and many minerals—all are important for your health and your baby's health.[6] What's not to like about all that, right? Well, don't get too excited just yet. If we take into consideration a person's existing health status and individual food sensitivities, also referred to as biochemical individuality, what is good for one person isn't necessarily good for another, especially if one of them is pregnant.

Keeping weight gain under control is critical to a healthy pregnancy, but so is maintaining stable blood sugar levels. A starchy vegetable like potatoes can contribute to both of those health issues, so for many people this becomes more important than the nutrients they contribute to your body.

The high amount of starch found in potatoes makes them a high-glycemic food. (Starch turns into sugar when digested.) Negatives with some foods, like potatoes, also have to do with how it is prepared. Most people understand that french fries are usually steeped in hydrogenated fats, which make them a bad food choice for everyone, including pregnant moms.

But there are also other biochemical disadvantages. Potatoes are considered to be part of the nightshade family of vegetables; they contain steroid alkaloids that can be inflammatory and alter mineral status in people with nerve-related conditions or arthritis.[7] They also contain solanine, which slows the production of important enzymes in the body (acetylcholinesterase), which are needed for mom and baby to have healthy nerves and muscles.[8] A small amount of potato—baked, boiled, or steamed—is probably not going to hurt you while pregnant. But if you're loading up on them three to five times a week and eating other starchy, high carb/sugary foods, then you could be setting yourself up for problems.

I really picked on potatoes here, but they are an excellent example of the type of nuances a food can have that makes an otherwise healthy food become a poor choice during pregnancy.

Because of some of these nuances with various foods, I am providing you with comprehensive details of what foods are good for you, which ones to minimize in your daily diet, and the ones that should be removed from your kitchen, never again to be seen on your grocery list—pre- or post-pregnancy.

Please familiarize yourself with the detailed information that follows. You don't want to "wing it" when it comes to your food choices, and take it from me as a former sugar addict, you definitely don't want to go with what you're craving on a given day.

Let's Talk about Weight Gain

When I was pregnant, I would be climbing the nursery room walls if I didn't get a chocolate brownie sundae every day. Between the horrific amount of weight I gained and the big ugly tent dresses that were fashionable back then, I looked enormous, bloated, and horribly unhealthy by the time I was barely eight months pregnant. If only I had known then what I know now about nutrition, I could have spared myself, my daughter, and my granddaughter from being genetically wired for insulin resistance and a whole laundry list of related health issues.

Ignorance is *not* bliss when you're pregnant. Being informed is empowering. Effective use of information gets you results, so please keep reading.

When it comes to weight gain during pregnancy, some women become fanatical about watching their weight. Then there are others who decide to eat whatever they want and let nature run its course. In many cases with the latter approach, nature is going to run you right into Problemville if you don't pay attention (as it did with me). Weight gain during pregnancy will put you at risk for pregnancy-related hypertension, preeclampsia (damage to organs can occur from hypertension), gestational diabetes, complications during labor and delivery, postpartum weight retention, and postpartum obesity.[9] The extra weight causes lots of concern well beyond the normal worries about losing all of it after your baby is delivered.

Adequate, normal weight gain during pregnancy is a determining factor for normal fetal development, which is an important reason why most healthcare practitioners will monitor it closely. During the first trimester when your fetus is very, very small and just beginning its developmental journey, weight gain is not expected or needed.[10] It is during the second and third trimesters that a steady weight gain of three to four pounds each month is recommended.

The current weight-gain guidelines during pregnancy were developed by the Institute of Medicine and re-evaluated in 2009 due to the significant changes that have occurred among the female population in their child-bearing years.[11] According to the IOM, American women are a more diverse group then they were two decades ago when IOM's original weight gain recommendations were developed. For instance, twin and triplet pregnancies are more common, which of course changes nutrition and weight requirements. Another key distinction is that women tend to be older when they become pregnant.[12] Women today also weigh more; they are often overweight or obese at the time of conception and are prone to excess weight gain during pregnancy.[13] Lastly, IOM's research acknowledges the added burden on women's health from the escalating frequency of chronic disease in the U.S., and the importance of dealing with existing health issues *prior to* becoming pregnant.[14]

As a result of these factors, weight gain recommendations are now based on the woman's pre-pregnancy body mass index, or BMI. As you will see in the IOM chart below, women who are underweight or normal weight prior to becoming pregnant will be expected to gain slightly more weight during their pregnancy than those who are overweight or obese.

To calculate your BMI, go to www.nhlbi.nih.gov/health/educationl/lose_wt/bmitools.htm.[15]

New Recommendations for Total and Rate of Weight Gain during Pregnancy, by Pre-pregnancy BMI*

Pre-pregnancy BMI	BMI Category	Total Weight Gain Range (in pounds)	Rate of Weight Gain During 2nd & 3rd Trimester (mean range in pounds/week)
Underweight	< 18.5	28 – 40	1 (1 – 1.3)
Normal weight	18.5 – 24.9	25 – 35	1 (0.8 – 1)
Overweight	25.0 – 29.9	15 – 25	0.6 (0.5 – 0.7)
Obese	>30.0	11 – 20	0.5 (0.4 – 0.6)

Source: Institute of Medicine, National Research Council. (2009) *Weight gain during pregnancy: Reexaming the guidelines.* National Academies Press. Washington, DC, accessed 4-26-17 at www.nationalacademies.org

Calculations assume a 1.1–4.4-pound weight gain in the first trimester (based on Siega-Riz et al., 1994; Abrams et al., 1995; Carmichael et al., 1997).

Food Cravings

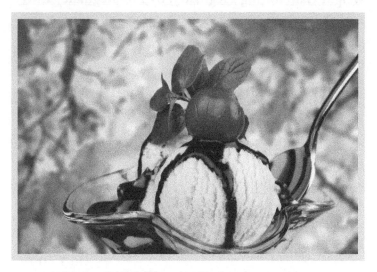

Source: StockAdobe.com. Used with permission.

With a lot of women, following your cravings will lead you directly to your local ice cream shop or Godiva chocolate store. I gave you a little insight about my experience with cravings in the previous section. I was like an addict during my pregnancy, and chocolate was my drug. I *needed* it. Unfortunately for me, I had an obstetrician who just shrugged his shoulders and didn't think much of it. Or maybe he saw the crazed look on my face as I described the new food group I discovered (chocolate). I'm sure I gave him scary visions of a chocolate-crazed pregnant woman strangling him with his stethoscope. Whatever the reason, he decided not to go there, and I conveniently interpreted his indifference as a glowing approval of my food choices. You might be able to fool (or, in my case, frighten) your doctor into silence, but you and your baby will face the potential health consequences. Make informed choices.

The typical food cravings during pregnancy include things like chocolate, sugary foods, spicy foods, pickles, potato chips, fruit, and ice cream. Simply caving to these demands on a regular basis will make you susceptible to excess weight gain during your pregnancy, and this puts your health and your baby's health at risk.

There are a small number of women who report cravings for non-nutritive substances, which is called pica and most often seen in children, to a lesser extent in pregnant women.[16] (The word "pica" is Latin for magpie, which is a bird notorious for eating almost anything.) There is not a definitive cause for why pica occurs during pregnancy for some women, but iron-deficiency has suspected involvement. Eight percent to 65 percent of pregnant women dealing with pica cravings will actually give in to them and consume the substance they crave.[17] The most common are dirt, clay, and laundry starch, but other known substances include):[18]

- Burnt matches
- Stones
- Charcoal
- Mothballs
- Ice
- Cornstarch
- Toothpaste
- Soap
- Sand
- Plaster
- Coffee grounds
- Baking soda

Nearly everything on this list is potentially harmful to you and your baby and should be avoided. Consuming any of these substances can interfere with absorption of much-needed nutrients, can cause other deficiencies, and may contain toxic ingredients. If you find yourself craving non-nutritive substances, it is important to notify your doctor or healthcare practitioner so you can be evaluated for a possible deficiency.

Making informed choices and decisions during your pregnancy includes knowing the things to avoid—things that can cause harm to you or your pregnancy. These topics are therefore covered separately in Chapter 7.

Blood Sugar, Glycemic Index, and Gestational Diabetes

Are you a sugar addict?

People don't want to admit they're addicts. In fact, they might not be aware their bodies are addicted to a substance. This is further complicated by a substance like sugar because a lot of people don't believe it is something that can cause addiction. Surprise! It most definitely can.

If you have a diet that is high in sugary fruits, soda or diet soda, breads, cakes, cookies, muffins, bagels, pasta, potatoes, rice, and processed and fast foods, then you also have a higher-than-average chance of being overweight. Also likely is that at some point in your life, you will experience what most people refer to as low blood sugar, or hypoglycemia. Basically, you're addicted to sugar. More specifically, this type of hypoglycemia is referred to as reactive hypoglycemia because it usually occurs three to five hours after eating a meal that is high in refined carbohydrates.[19]

Because glucose is the primary fuel for the brain, being hypoglycemic affects the brain first; it is the first organ to react to being depleted of fuel. Symptoms can be mild or severe and include dizziness, shakiness, hunger, headaches, irritability, pounding heart or racing pulse, sweating, trembling, weakness, or anxiety. Without treatment or immediately ingesting food (Usually the most relief will come from eating protein.), these symptoms can progress to numbness in the mouth and tongue, poor coordination, poor concentration, or even passing out.[20]

Hypoglycemia and its more advanced, wicked sister, diabetes, are becoming more common in the U.S., as are obesity and gestational diabetes. This shouldn't be a big surprise to anyone, given the average person in the U.S. consumes more than one hundred pounds of sucrose and forty pounds of high-fructose corn syrup (both are sugary substances) every year.[21]

Gestational Diabetes—What Is It?

There are many complications that can occur during pregnancy. Of these, gestational diabetes is one of the most common, and its incidence is on the rise. It brings with it considerable health risks to the mother and sometimes her baby. It is also a condition that, in most cases, can easily be avoided by paying attention to your diet. Since *Baby Maker* is all about nutrition, I wanted to take the time to cover this important, damaging, and easily avoidable condition.

Before I discuss the effects of gestational diabetes, you should understand how it occurs and who is at risk for it.

It is normal for blood glucose levels to rise a little during pregnancy, but if the mother's levels get too high, it starts to become a hazard to the health of mom and her baby, and this is when gestational diabetes will be diagnosed.

Blood glucose levels naturally become elevated when a women is pregnant because the placenta produces hormones (called "human placental lactogen" or HPL) that change the mother's metabolism and how she processes carbohydrates and fats.[22] The HPL raises the mother's blood glucose level, which makes her body less sensitive to insulin and less able to properly use it. If the body isn't using insulin as it should, then blood glucose levels will rise. In the second trimester, other hormones also increase, such as growth hormone, progesterone, cortisol, and prolactin—all of which contribute to a decrease in mom's insulin sensitivity and a rise in blood glucose level, and all by design to make sure the baby gets enough nutrients from the extra glucose in the blood.[23]

With all that extra glucose floating around in your bloodstream, controlling your intake of sugary foods becomes a critical component in supporting the body's natural ability to regulate blood sugar levels. Adding high-glycemic foods into the equation sets you up for problems.

Risk Factors and Affects

The risk factors for gestational diabetes are:

- Age: women over the age of twenty-five
- Weight: women who are overweight, a BMI at or around twenty-five
- Family history: someone else in the family has had diabetes (type 1, type 2, or gestational diabetes)

- Pre-diabetic: women who are pre-diabetic at conception. Being pre-diabetic means your blood glucose level is high but not high enough to be considered a diabetic. Being pre-diabetic is a high-risk factor for gestational diabetes.[24]

Previous pregnancy with gestational diabetes. If you had it in a previous pregnancy, you are likely to develop it in future pregnancies.

Here's how gestational diabetes can affect your baby at birth or right after birth:

- Excess growth (macrosomia). May cause your baby to put on extra weight and be very large at birth. This can make delivery more difficult, possibly requiring a C-section to deliver safely.[25]
- Low blood glucose (hypoglycemia). Your baby will have excess insulin in its body in response to the excess glucose in yours. Once the baby is delivered, the extra insulin can cause its blood sugar level to drop rapidly requiring medical intervention.[26]
- Difficulty breathing (respiratory distress syndrome). Breathing difficulties in babies occurs from time to time, but is more common when the mother has gestational diabetes. When the lungs become stronger, the breathing issues usually clear up.[27]

The risks don't end after the baby is no longer a newborn. Gestational diabetes can affect your child later in life as well. Children born from a mother diagnosed with gestational diabetes are at a higher risk for developmental problems and for developing type 2 diabetes later in life.[28]

The Silver Lining to Gestational Diabetes

Here's the silver lining with gestational diabetes: you can *dramatically* minimize your risk of this ever occurring by making dietary changes several months *before* getting pregnant, adding regular moderate exercise to your routine three to five times a week, and getting your weight and blood sugar at healthy levels.

What Is the Glycemic Index?

A major first step in avoiding the health challenges of gestational diabetes and putting on too much weight during pregnancy is learning which foods are okay to eat, which ones aren't, which foods are high in sugar, and which ones aren't. There are also foods that are low in sugar but have compounds that cause insulin to be produced when they are digested. Too much sugar and/or too much insulin production and you are setting yourself up for gestational diabetes.

You have to gain insight into how *your* body reacts to carbohydrates and sugar. If you are overweight, feel like you gain weight easily, and/or have issues with blood sugar regulation (blood sugar drops after eating), those are all indications that your body is not metabolizing glucose properly. You will want to correct this now, well before trying to conceive.

There is a handy rating system for food that was developed by a research professor in 1981, originally to benefit diabetics. It is called the Glycemic Index (GI) and Glycemic Load (GL).[29] Over time, nutrition and diet experts used the GI concept to test hundreds of foods in a laboratory setting, the results of which were compiled to form the Glycemic Index Chart.

As we discussed in the previous section, sugar—or glucose—is the body's main source of energy for many biological activities. Without it we would all be dragging our worn-out bodies around, unable to think clearly, move around fluidly, or even climb a short flight of stairs. Sugar is a necessary fuel source. It is delivered throughout the body to cells via our bloodstream that most typically come from the carbohydrates in the foods we eat. You will often hear of athletes using a "carb-loading" diet to boost energy, endurance, and stamina.

The problem many people make—athletes and non-athletes—is in thinking that *all* sugar and *all* carbohydrates are beneficial to the body. Just not true, and this is where the Glycemic Index can be helpful.

The GI Scale

The GI uses a scale of 1 to 100 to rate foods on how fast and how high different foods raises blood sugar levels, with one being virtually no increase and one hundred being the highest. Foods that are digested and absorbed faster will usually be rated seventy or higher on the index. Fifty-five and under is considered low GI, while fifty-six to sixty-nine is a medium rating. In other words, the GI ratings given to a carbohydrate provide an accurate description of how quickly it will be absorbed by the body, more accurate than anyone can determine just by looking at how many grams of sugar on a food label or knowing if it is a "simple" or "complex" carbohydrate.[30]

A food with a low GI (under fifty-five) causes a small increase in blood glucose, but a food with a high GI (over seventy) can cause a rapid spike that more often than not will be very noticeable to the individual.[31]

Low GI: 55 and under
Medium GI: 56 to 69
High GI: 70 and above
(Mateljan, 2007)

Eating the Low-Glycemic Way

Healthy women who are planning to conceive or who are already pregnant should consume only minimal amounts of high-GI foods; try to limit them to one small serving a day. Women who are hypoglycemic, insulin resistant, overweight or diabetic before conception need to completely avoid high GI foods *and* limit the amount of medium GI foods to no more than one small serving a day, both prior to conception and throughout the pregnancy.

Here are a few other guidelines to help you figure out a food's Glycemic Index rating and stay on track with a low-sugar, healthy diet:

- Foods that are white tend to have a high GI. These would include processed foods made with white sugar or white flour, as well as white potatoes.
- Concentrate on eating foods that are high in fiber. High-fiber foods take longer to digest and therefore produce a slower rise in blood glucose levels.
- Protein foods, while not high in fiber, are typically low in GI.
- Fats do not raise glucose levels, but focus on healthy fats such as those found in organic butter, organic extra virgin olive oil, wild-caught fish, and unsalted/unroasted nuts and seeds.

By eating a wide variety of nutrient-rich foods each day will you maintain a healthy GI. Your glycemic response to a food not only depends upon the other foods you eat along with it at that meal or snack, but also on the GI of foods eaten at other recent meals.

Now, for those of you who are really paying attention, this does not give you permission to eat as much sugary junk food as you want as long as you have a broccoli chaser with it each time. But for those of you who are healthy prior to conception, not dealing with insulin resistance, obesity, hypoglycemia, or other health issues, it gives you the flexibility of including a small amount of high-glycemic foods without having to worry about blood sugar issues. In other words, your body should be able to handle a small dessert once a day without worrying about sugar-overload.

An awareness of a foods' rating can help you control your blood sugar levels, which in turn can help you avoid many health issues, including some cancers, heart disease, insulin resistance, and gestational diabetes.[32] I strongly encourage you to become familiar with the GI list of foods below. This is not a comprehensive list by any means, and ratings can vary slightly depending on the formula used to calculate them, but this will give you a good idea of how commonly consumed foods are rated and help you make healthier food choices during your pregnancy.[33]

I encourage wannabe moms to photocopy this list or write out your own list of glycemic ratings for the foods you like to eat. Keep it with you for a while until you get a handle on your daily sugar intake and how much your food intake is contributing to it.

Food List—Glycemic Index Rating

Vegetables	Rating
Spinach	15
Turnip Greens	15
Lettuce	15
Watercress	15
Zucchini	15
Asparagus	15
Artichokes	15
Okra	15
Cabbage	15
Cucumbers	15
Dill Pickles	15
Radishes	15
Broccoli	15
Brussel sprouts	15
Eggplant	15
Onions	15
Tomatoes	15
Cauliflower	30
Bell peppers	40
Green Peas	40
Carrots	47
Squash	50
Sweet potatoes	61
Beet root	64
French fries	75
Pumpkin	75
Broad beans	79
Baked potato	85
Parsnips	97

Grains	
Bagel	69
Baguette	57

Barley, cooked	35
Barley kernel bread	64
Barley flour bread	94
Whole meal barley porridge	95
Buckwheat bread	66
Buckwheat, cooked	76
Corn, yellow	78
Corn tortillas	78
Corn flakes	77
Taco shells	97
Millet, boiled	99
Multi-grain bread	79
Oat bran bread	66
Oatmeal (instant)	92
Muesli	80
Rice bread	72
Rye bread	50

Fruits

Apples	53
Apricots	80
Banana, ripe	73
Dried dates	103
Grapefruit	35
Grapes	64
Kiwi	74
Oranges	59
Papaya	83
Peach	42
Pear	53
Cantaloupe	91
Strawberries	56
Watermelon	100

(Mateljan, 2007)

Healthy Eating by Food Group

If you're officially eating for two or will be soon, this means your body needs more of everything in order to have adequate levels to support your health and your baby's health. It requires more calories, protein, calcium, iron, zinc, B vitamins, essential fatty acids, most other vitamins, and minerals, and it needs more time for rest as well as continued exercise and movement.

Below you will find details on how some of the major food groups contribute to a healthy diet for pregnancy. These are mostly foods you will want to increase in your daily diet, along with serving sizes and nutrient content information to help you make smart decisions. Many of these food groups require increased daily amounts during lactation as well as pregnancy, which is outlined in the post-pregnancy health issues covered in Chapter 8. Each food category includes a "daily recommendation during pregnancy." The categories and recommendations are summarized for you at the end of the chapter.

Once again, please refer back to the visual depiction of your daily diet, "My Holistic Pregnancy Plate" found earlier in this chapter. Note that grains are combined in the same food group as starchy vegetables and there is not a separate group for dairy. Grains and starchy vegetables both contain relatively high amounts of carbohydrates, i.e., sugar, which should not be our nutritional focus if we want to sustain good health, especially during pregnancy. I'll explain more about this in subsequent pages.

<u>Dairy</u>

First of all, dairy is actually a protein, so if we were going to include it in a dietary plan it would be part of the protein food group. However, my hope is that you eliminate dairy completely, or consume it only in small quantities, and here's why. Dairy products are known to be highly inflammatory, acid-forming foods, causing digestive issues such as bloating, gas, constipation, diarrhea, acne outbreaks, and even autistic behaviors in some individuals.[34] The acidic nature of dairy foods will cause an imbalance in your internal pH, causing your body to compensate for the increased acidity.[35] It does this by drawing on the alkaline "reserves" in the body, which means calcium, magnesium, and potassium are pulled out of your bones to rebalance your pH.[36] In addition, dairy products often contain hormones and antibiotics since most livestock that produces milk is injected with these chemical substances.

We were all taught that milk helps build strong bones, but unfortunately, consuming it in excess during pregnancy might work against you. Your goal is to minimize inflammation and maintain a healthy, neutral internal pH in the body. If you're worried about where you will get your calcium, don't. Calcium is found in foods such as almonds, kale, collard greens, broccoli, spinach, almond, hemp and coconut milks, and sesame seeds. In addition, calcium will either be in your prenatal vitamin or will be on your individualized supplement list.

The Role of Fats in Pregnancy

Eating adequate amounts of healthy fats is critical to a healthy pregnancy. Look at it this way: you can't build a new house without a solid foundation, right? You also can't have a healthy pregnancy and baby without healthy fats; they are the building blocks of the human body. They are required for a healthy immune system, the absorption of fat-soluble vitamins, regulation of blood sugar and blood clotting, and they are a major source of energy.[37]

They play a vital role in reproduction and pregnancy as well. Fats are critical to fetal brain and retina development. They play a role in determining the length of gestation, preventing perinatal depression and contribute to normal growth and maturation of fetal organ systems.[38]

Some people will wrinkle their noses at me when I tell them to eat more high-quality fats, which is understandable given the number of years our food regulators and governments agencies have warned us of the perils of a high-fat diet. But the truth is, not all fats are harmful. In fact, healthy fats, including cholesterol, are fundamental to good health. The key to unlocking the paradox we've been living with all these years is in understanding the difference between good fats and bad fats. There are very lengthy books written about fats (also known as lipids) that would put your newborn baby to sleep real fast if you were to read it out loud. Lucky for you, I'm not going to get into that level of detail, but will try to explain, briefly, what you need to know.

More on Fats

There are three types of healthy fats (fatty acids): saturated, monounsaturated, and polyunsaturated. Of these, polyunsaturated contain a special subgroup called essential fatty acids. They are considered "essential" fatty acids (EFAs) because they cannot be produced by the body but are required for healthy bodily functions. They must be obtained from foods or supplements. The active forms of these fats are docosahexaenoic acid (DHA) and eicosapentaenoic acid (EPA), and are primarily found in seafood, algae, and fish-oil supplements.[39]

There are two main families of essential fatty acids, which you might recognize: omega-3 and omega-6. As mentioned previously, these EFAs are required for physiologic functions in the body such as energy storage, cell membrane function, regulation of inflammation (infection) and healthy cell growth.[40]

When you read anything at all about fats, it's typical to conclude that omega-3 fats are "good" and omega-6 fats are "bad." This is incorrect. We actually need both, but the focus needs to be on keeping them balanced. In fact, the human body needs a healthy, balanced ratio of omega-3 to omega-6, ideally 1:1, one gram of omega-3s for every gram of omega-6 fats.[41] This ratio is not easy to achieve, however. The current average ratio in the U.S. is estimated at 15:1 but goes as high as 45:1 in some people.[42] If your diet consists of a lot of fried foods, processed foods, and meals from fast food restaurants, it's very likely your ratio is in line with the rest of America, which means your focus needs to be on increasing the amount of omega 3 fats in your diet in order to support your body and the developing baby inside you.[43] Without the proper ratio of omega-3 to omega-6 fats, you increase the risk of preterm labor and preeclampsia, along with fetal developmental issues.[44]

The omega-3 fats we hear about most often relating to pregnancy are known as EPA and DHA. They are both derived from their "parent" fatty acid which is a-linolenic acid or ALA. ALA is converted to EPA, which eventually gets converted to DHA in the body.[45] DHA becomes the critical fatty acid for brain and retina development, as well as neurotransmitter metabolism. Because the human body is not very efficient at converting ALA to DHA and, as already mentioned, most of us in the U.S. have an imbalance of the necessary fatty acids, we most often see only DHA represented in prenatal fish-oil supplements.[46]

Dos and Don'ts of Fats[47]

- Do eat healthy fats (not damaged fats).
- Do purchase high-quality, organic butter and oils.
- Do eat fresh food containing fats and keep refrigerated.
- Do keep monounsaturated and polyunsaturated oils in opaque, airtight containers to prevent oxidation (damage to fat molecules).
- Do read labels to avoid buying fats that contain added chemicals.
- Do cook fatty meats at low temperatures to avoid oxidation (damage to fat molecules).
- Don't cook with polyunsaturated oils (safflower, grapeseed, sunflower, walnut, soybean, corn, and cottonseed oils).
- Don't cook with butter at high temperatures. Butter contains polyunsaturated oils and can be damaged with high heat. (Ghee, or clarified butter that has the milk solids removed, is best choice for cooking.)
- Don't use low-fat or nonfat products. They are not whole foods and are not healthier for you. Most have the fats removed and replaced with sugar or other artificial chemicals.
- Don't eat foods high in fat by themselves. It's best to avoid them altogether, but if you can't resist the order of greasy french fries, at least eat them with a serving of vegetables or a salad.

- Don't eat too much or too little fat. Doing so will damage your metabolism and can cause harm to fertility and reproduction, fetal brain and retina development, as well as fetal cell membrane structure.[48]

Food Sources of Omega-3 Fatty Acids

Foods that are high in omega-3 fats are listed below. As most people know, seafood is an excellent source of omega-3 fatty acids, so I would like to make special mention of it here.

In spite of seafood being packed full of good healthy fats, many women who otherwise love to eat fish will avoid it completely during pregnancy. This is due primarily to fears that seafood has high mercury content and other heavy metals, as published by the Food and Drug Administration (FDA) and the Environmental Protection Agency (EPA).[49] But even the FDA and EPA recognize the importance of having fats in the diet and suggest two servings (about twelve ounces) of seafood per week is adequate during pregnancy.[50]

While the warnings about the mercury content of seafood should be taken seriously, you should also take very seriously the need to have adequate omega-3 fats in your diet. For this reason my recommendations are to take advantage of the high omega-3 content of seafood by eating it up to three times per week, but use care to avoid the critters that are most often contaminated. For more information about this important topic, see Chapter 7.

If you enjoy eating fish, the key is to buy high-quality, wild-caught and consume species such as wild salmon, sardines, and small mackerel to minimize exposure to heavy metals. These fish do not accumulate mercury, while tuna, for example, is a moderate mercury accumulator. If you are like me and can't stand being near someone who is eating fish, much less eat it yourself, you need to get your omega fats from a good nutritional supplement and other food sources.

Daily recommendations during pregnancy:

- Get 20 to 35 percent of your total caloric intake from quality fat sources. (Refer to food lists in Chapter 4.)
- Focus intake on foods high in omega-3 fats.[51]
- Limit seafood intake to wild-caught only, two to three servings per week. Avoid types of fish known to be high in mercury and other toxins (shellfish, shark, swordfish, king mackerel, tilefish, marlin, orange roughy, and tuna).[52]
- Include a high-quality EPA/DHA fish-oil supplement with your supplement regimen.

Food sources of Omega-3 Fatty Acids (cont.)

Food	Serving Size	Omega-3 Content (g)
FISH		
Fatty fish: *wild-caught salmon, sardines, mackerel or albacore tuna, bluefish*[53]	4 ounces	0.3 – 2.1
Medium-fat fish: *trout, rockfish, oysters, mussels*[54]	4 ounces	0.5 – 0.8
Low-fat fish: *halibut, crab, cod, clams, flounder, scallops, lobster, sole, orange roughy, shrimp*[55]	4 ounces	0.1 – 0.4
MEAT		
Lamb	3 ½ ounces	0.5
Beef, poultry	3 ½ ounces	0.2
OILS		
Flax oil	1 Tbsp	6.6
Flax meal	1 Tbsp	1.6
Canola oil	1 Tbsp	1.6
NUTS AND SEEDS		
Walnuts	2 Tbsp	1.0
Chia seeds	2 Tbsp	1.1
LEGUMES AND TOFU		
Soybeans, cooked	1 cup	1.1
Tofu, firm	4 ounces	0.4
VEGETABLES		
Broccoli, kale, leafy greens	1 cup	0.1
Cauliflower	1 cup	0.2
Brussels Sprouts	1 cup	0.3
Winter Squash	1 cup	0.3
Summer Squash	1 cup	0.2
Green Beans	1 cup	0.1

Food Sources of Omega-6 Fatty Acids

Daily recommendation for omega-6 fats during pregnancy:

- Avoid using fats and oils high in omega-6

Food	Serving Size	Omega-6 (g)
PLANT FOODS		
FATS AND OILS		
Safflower oil	1 Tbsp	10.0
Sunflower oil	1 Tbsp	9.0
Corn oil	1 Tbsp	8.0
Soybean oil	1 Tbsp	7.0
Peanut oil	1 Tbsp	4.5
Canola oil	1 Tbsp	2.5
Mayonnaise	1 Tbsp	5.0
NUTS AND SEEDS		
(best if sprouted)	¼ cup	9.0
Sesame, pumpkin, sunflower seeds	1 ounce	4.0
Peanuts, walnuts, Brazil, pine nuts	1 ounce	2.0
Almonds, cashews, pecans, hazelnuts		
LEGUMES AND WHOLE GRAINS		
Legumes	½ cup	0.2
Wheat germ	2 Tbsp	1.0
Grains (wheat, rice, oats, and so forth)	½ cup cooked	0.5

VEGEATABLES AND FRUITS

Avocado	1 whole	3.5
All others	½ cup or 1 medium fruit	0.05

MEAT AND FISH

Poultry (light and dark meat)	3 ½ ounces	2.0
Pork (lean)	3 ½ ounces	0.7
Beef (lean)	3 ½ ounces	0.3
Fish (high-fat varieties)	3 ½ ounces	0.2
Fish (low-fat varieties)	3 ½ ounces	0.1

Recommended Oils and Fats

Use mostly monounsaturated oils and some saturated fats. Use polyunsaturated oils sparingly or not all. When using them, choose pure-pressed, cold-pressed, or expeller-pressed.

Monounsaturated	Polyunsaturated	Saturated
Almond oil	Corn oil	Most other
Apricot kernel oil	Cottonseed oil	vegetable oils
Avocado oil	Essential fatty acids	Butter
Canola oil	(borage, flaxseed,	Cheese
Hazelnut oil	primrose)	Chicken fat
Mustard oil	Herring oil	Coconut oil
Oat oil	Menhaden (fish) oil	Cream
Olive oil	Safflower oil	Duck fat
Peanut oil	Salmon oil	Eggs
Rice oil	Sardine oil	Ghee
Most nuts	Sesame oil	(clarified butter)
Most other nut oils	Soybean oil	Meats
	Sunflower oil	Nutmeg oil
	Wheat germ oil	Shea nut oil
		Turkey fat

Recommended Oils and Fats

- Extra-virgin olive oil
- Cold-, pure-, or expeller-pressed vegetable oils (not good for cooking)
- Essential fatty acids—primrose, flaxseed, salmon, borage (Do not cook with these oils.)

Mayonnaise that is made from avocado oil or other cold-, pure-, or expeller-pressed oil and contains neither hydrogenated nor partially hydrogenated oils.

Protein Foods That Contain Carbohydrates

Nuts, nut butters, and seeds are great sources of protein, omega-3 essential fatty acids, and healthy monounsaturated fats such as oleic acid and other nutrients. Because of their broad nutrient content, nuts and seeds are an excellent choice if you're looking for a snack. However, be aware that most of them are also high in calories so you will want to limit your daily intake to one or two small handfuls a day during pregnancy. Like other foods, it is important to check the ingredient label when choosing nuts and seeds to watch for unwanted ingredients. Honey-roasted nuts are coated in sugar, and cashews are frequently covered in peanut oil, which is high in pro-inflammatory omega-6 fats.[56] Foods that contain carbohydrates should also be checked against the Glycemic Index ratings to keep blood sugar levels low.

Food	Serving
Acorns	½ ounce
Almonds	1 ounce (23 nuts)
Almond butter	4 tablespoons
Almond paste	½ ounce
Amaranth seed	⅓ ounce
Brazil nuts (butternuts)	1 ½ ounces
Cashews	¾ ounce
Cashew butter	1 ½ tablespoons
Chinese chestnuts	½ ounce
Coconut cream	¼ cup
Coconut liquid from coconut	¾ cup
Coconut meat	½ cup
Coconut milk	½ cup
Cottonseed kernels	1 ounce
European chestnuts	½ ounce
Hazelnuts	1 ½ ounces
Ginkgo nuts	½ ounce
Hickory nuts	1 ounce
Japanese chestnuts	¾ ounce
Lotus seeds	1 ½ ounces
Macadamia nuts	1 ounce
Peanuts (organic)	1 ounce
Peanut butter (organic)	2 tablespoons
Pecans	1 ounce (15 halves)
Pine nuts	1 ounce
Pistachio nuts	1 ounce (47 kernels)
Pumpkin and squash kernels	1 ounce
Pumpkin and squash seeds	½ ounce (42 seeds)
Safflower kernels	½ ounce
Sesame butter	1 ½ tablespoons
Sesame seeds	1 ounce
Sunflower seed butter	1 ½ tablespoons
Sunflower seeds	¼ cup
Walnuts	2 ounces
Watermelon seeds	⅜ cup

Yogurt

Each of the following serving sizes contains approximately 15 grams of carbohydrates.

Food Item	Serving
Plain whole-milk yogurt, cow	1 cup
Plain whole-milk yogurt, goat	1 cup
Plain whole-milk yogurt, Indian buffalo	1 cup
Plain whole-milk yogurt, sheep	1 cup
Soy yogurt	1 cup

Gluten-Free Grains

Most people believe a gluten-free diet is only necessary for those diagnosed with celiac disease. Like many practitioners in holistic nutrition or functional medicine, I recommend a gluten-free diet to all my clients, especially when dealing with fertility issues, pregnancy, or other chronic health conditions. It is a trouble-causing, pro-inflammatory substance that most of us can and should do without.

Gluten is made up of two groups of proteins, the glutenins and the gliadins, which are the proteins found in wheat, barley, and rye. Due to the sticky properties of these two proteins, they are commonly used in pastas, noodles, breads, pastries, crackers, baked goods, cereals, croutons, sauces, and beer—to name just a few sources. (See Appendix for list of products containing gluten.) Both are known to cause a range of reaction in the body from celiac disease (an autoimmune response to gluten), to a non-celiac wheat sensitivity, or a non-celiac sensitivity.[57]

In his book, *Grain Brain*, Doctor David Perlmutter describes celiac disease as "an extreme manifestation of gluten sensitivity."[58] He estimates 1 in 30 people is affected with celiac disease, with a large number of these yet to be diagnosed.[59]

Doctor Perlmutter goes on to describe typical reactions to gluten:

> "The key to understanding gluten sensitivity is that it can involve any organ in the body, even if the small intestine is completely spared. So while a person may not have celiac disease by definition, the rest of the body—including the brain—is at great risk if that individual is gluten sensitive."[60]

In the context of this book, the significance to the widespread, internal, damaging effects of gluten is that it is also tied to unexplained infertility and miscarriage.

Signs and symptoms of celiac disease include:

- Gastrointestinal—pain, bloating, gas, constipation or diarrhea, loss of appetite, nausea, vomiting
- Brain and nervous system—recurring headaches, decreased sensation in peripheral nerves, anxiety, panic attacks, depression. Other bodily systems—fatigue, itchy, skin rash, unexplained infertility and miscarriage, arthritis, iron-deficiency anemia, and other nutritional deficiencies.[61]

There are some differences in symptoms with non-celiac sensitivity, but not enough to throw all caution to the wind and give you the green light to eat gluten just because you are not diagnosed with celiac disease. Our goal in cleaning up your diet is to eliminate foods and lifestyle choices that cause inflammation and may contribute to infertility or health issues related to your pregnancy. The bottom line is that gluten causes a production of pro-inflammatory chemicals that wreak havoc in the gastrointestinal system and elsewhere in the body.

With your focus now on gluten-free grains, you can take comfort in the fact that even gluten-free whole grains can provide a wide range of important nutrients. These include dietary fiber; vitamin E; vitamin B complex; minerals such as magnesium, iron, and zinc; and plenty of phytonutrients (plant nutrients). Grains found in processed foods (such as bagels, cookies, cakes, or multi-grain bread), not only contain gluten, but typically have the nutrient-dense germ bran stripped away, leaving a starchy complex carbohydrate that basically fills you up with sugar, leaving you feeling like your blood sugar is on a roller-coaster ride. To get the benefits of these nutrients, you must consume whole grains that contain the germ and bran, which is where the nutrients are found. When combined the grain is also, lower on the glycemic index.. Grains need to be chosen carefully and consumed in small quantities, even if gluten-free. Check food labels for additives and sugar content.

Daily recommendations:

- Choose products that are made with gluten-free grains (listed below).
- Limit intake to maximum of two servings per day, gluten-free only.
- If blood sugar issues are present or other health concerns, limit gluten-free grains to no more than three times per week.

Each of the following gluten-free serving sizes contains about fifteen grams of carbohydrates.

Food Item	Serving
Amaranth	⅓ cup
Brown rice	⅓ cup
Buckwheat (whole-grain)	⅓ cup
Buckwheat groats (kasha)	⅓ cup
Cornmeal (whole grain)	¼ cup
Millet	⅓ cup
Oats	⅓ cup
Polenta	⅓ cup
Popcorn	2 ¼ cup
Quinoa	⅓ cup
Sorghum	¼ cup
Teff	¼ cup
Wild rice	½ cup

Gluten-Free Whole-Grain Flour and Meals

Each of the following serving sizes contains approximately fifteen grams of carbohydrates.

All items are dry.

Food Item	Serving
Almond meal	½ cup
Amaranth flour	2 Tbsp
Arrowroot flour	2 Tbsp
Brown rice flour	2 Tbsp
Buckwheat flour (whole-grain)	3 ½ Tbsp
Pecan flour	¾ cup
Potato flour	1 ½ Tbsp
Sesame flour	2 ½ Tbsp
Soy flour	½ cup
Sunflower seed flour	¼ cup
Sesame flour	1 ½ ounces

<u>Protein</u>

Proteins are often recognized as one of the most important nutrients in the human body. They account for 20 percent of our body weight and perform a wide range of functions, especially during pregnancy.[62]

The body manufactures proteins, mainly from amino acids, which are the building blocks of all proteins. Once proteins are formed in the body, they are used to create hair, muscles, nails, tendons, ligaments, brain, blood, and other body structures. They also function as enzymes, hormones, and important parts of other cells, such as our genes.[63] Because proteins are the foundation of all bodily tissues and many functions, a deficiency during pregnancy can create significant risk to a developing fetus, including premature birth, poor muscular and skeletal development, low birth rate, and other health complications.[64]

Like other nutrients we cover in this book, the quality of a food makes an impact on how it is absorbed, stored and used in the body. A "complete" protein source is one that provides adequate amounts of all nine essential amino acids. But not all proteins are "complete." This is important to understand. The human body can manufacture most of the twenty amino acids it needs, but the nine that are "essential" can only be derived from the food you eat. This means what you eat and how much *matters*!

Scientists use biological value (BV) to assess and compare protein quality.[65] An example of biological values is listed below. This will help give you an idea of the different quality ratings of various foods.

Biological Value of Protein Sources[66]

Food	Biological Value (BV)
Whey protein concentrate	110–159
Whey protein	104
Egg protein	100
Whole egg	93.7
Milk	84.5
Fish	76
Beef	74.3
Rice, polished	64.0
Wheat, whole	64.0
Corn	60.0
Beans, dry	58.0

Daily dietary recommendations:

Protein amounts vary according to your weight. The average protein consumption is sixty to seventy-five grams of protein per day during the first trimester. See Chapter 5 for recommendations by trimester.

- Protein sources should be varied and include unsweetened hemp, coconut or almond milks, eggs, and high quality organic meats and fish.

Protein Portions

Two-Ounce Portions

Two ounces of protein is approximately half the size of your palm and as thick as a deck of cards. Examples of two-ounce protein portions include:

- 2 ounces beef, lamb, pork, chicken, turkey, or fish
- 2 eggs
- 2 ounces canned tuna (⅓ can)
- ½ cup cottage cheese
- 2 ounces cheese
- Nuts: 2 ounces almonds, 3 ounces other nuts

Three-Ounce Portions

Three ounces of protein is approximately the size and thickness of a deck of cards. Examples of three-ounce protein portions include:

- 3 ounces beef, lamb, pork, chicken, turkey, fish
- 3 eggs
- 3 ounces canned tuna (½ can)
- ¾ cup grass-fed cottage cheese
- 3 ounces grass-fed cheese

Four-Ounce Portions

Four ounces of protein is approximately the size of your palm and as thick as a deck of cards. Examples of 4 ounces protein portions include:

- 4 ounces beef, lamb, pork, chicken, turkey, fish
- 4 eggs
- 4 ounces canned tuna (⅔ can)
- 1 cup cottage cheese
- 4 ounces cheese (Try to limit cheese to 2 ounces unless you are a vegetarian.)

Eggs

Eggs are considered to be nearly a perfect food given the high quality of protein they provide, in addition to other vitamins and minerals. It is often the standard by which all other proteins are compared and rated.[67] Eat eggs every day, choose organic, and eat as many as your body wants.

Meat

Whenever possible, buy hormone-free, antibiotic-free, range-fed meat.

Beef*	Pheasant	Squab
Chicken**	Pork (bacon, ham)*	Turkey**
Duck*	Quail	Veal
Lamb*		

*Bacon and ham are often cured with sugar. If you must eat bacon or ham, only do so occasionally and always make sure you are buying nitrate-free meats. Beef, duck, and lamb contain glycogen, a hidden sugar. All contain saturated fats. Watch your portions if you are insulin-resistant.

**Dark chicken and turkey meat have more saturated fat. Eat mostly white meat, especially if you are insulin-resistant.

Vegetables (non-starchy)

Vegetables are rich in nutrients and low in calories, meaning they provide the most vitamins, minerals, and phytonutrients (plant nutrients) for the fewest number of calories when compared to other food groups. In fact, vegetables, along with fruits, are the most concentrated sources of health-promoting phytonutrients. During pre-conception, pregnancy and nursing, vegetables should make up the largest percentage of food consumed each day. The best way to incorporate vegetables into your diet is to eat them raw and to eat a variety. Foods almost always lose some nutrient value in the cooking process, especially considering that most people have a tendency to overcook vegetables, and this causes a substantial nutrient loss. If you are going to cook them, do so for a short time, just long enough to soften the outer portion—crisp on the inside, tender outside.

The exception to the "eat raw" recommendation has to do with cruciferous vegetables. At least minimal cooking time is recommended for cruciferous vegetables such as broccoli, cauliflower, arugula, brussels sprouts, cabbage, collard greens, and kale. Cruciferous vegetables contain compounds that are known as "goitrogens" and can cause disruption to the thyroid gland.[68]

Non-starchy vegetables are a source of fiber, vitamins, and minerals. The fiber slows the digestion and absorption of your carbohydrates, protein, and fats. This helps balance your hormones and at the same time allows only a small amount of the food to enter your bloodstream at any given moment. This is important because your body is able to process food more efficiently in smaller quantities. Fiber also helps add bulk to your bowel movements and is what your good bacteria use as food to thrive. This helps keep your colon healthy and happy. Vitamins and minerals found in non-starchy vegetables are used as coenzymes, which are chemicals that speed up biochemical reactions, and help you regenerate more efficiently.

BABY MAKER

Daily Vegetable Guidelines and Recommendations:

- Eat at least five servings or two and one-half cups of non-starchy vegetables a day and consume at least one serving with each meal, including breakfast.
- A portion of daily vegetable intake can be liquefied in a high-powered blender and consumed by drinking.
- Eat organically grown vegetables as much as possible to avoid pesticides and other toxins.[69]
- Vary your choices; different vegetables contain different antioxidants and phytochemicals that help keep you healthy.[70]
- You may eat frozen vegetables as long as there are no added preservatives or sugars. Watch out for hidden salt that may contribute to water-retention.
- Consider any vegetable that contains five or fewer grams of carbohydrates per half-cup serving to be a non-starchy vegetable.
- Limit intake of starchy vegetables to two servings per day. If blood sugar issues are present, starchy vegetables should be reduced to three or four servings a week.
- Carrots and tomatoes are considered both starchy and non-starchy vegetables. When you eat them raw, consider them non-starchy. When you cook them, consider them starchy. (Cooking breaks down fiber content.)

Non-Starchy Vegetables[71]

Serving sizes:

Cooked or raw vegetables	½ cup
Leafy green raw vegetables	1 cup
Vegetable juice	¾ cup
Fat-containing vegetables	¼ cup

Amaranth leaves
Arrowhead
Arugula
Asparagus
Balsam-pear
Bamboo shoots
Bean sprouts
Beet greens*
Bell peppers (red,
green, yellow)
Borage
Broadbeans
Broccoli
Brussels sprouts
Butterbur (fuki)
Cabbage
Carrots (raw)
Cassava
Cauliflower
Celeriac
Celery
Chayote fruit
Chicory greens
Chives
Chrysanthemum

Collard greens*
Coriander
Cowpeas (leafy tips)
Cucumber
Dandelion greens
Dock
Eggplant
Eppaw
Fennel
Gardencress
Garlic
Ginger root
Green beans
Heart of palm
Horseradish
Jalapeno peppers
Jute potherb
Kale*
Kohlrabi
Lamb's quarter
Lettuce
Mushrooms
Mustard greens
Onions Parsley
Pokeberry shoots

Pumpkin
flowers/leaves
Purslane
Radishes
Radicchio
Salsify
Scallop squash
Sesbania flower
Snap beans
Snow peas
Shallots
Spinach*
Spaghetti squash
Summer squash
Swiss chard*
Sweet peppers
Sweet potato leaves
Taro (leaves
or shoots)
Tomatoes (raw)
Tree fern
Turnip greens
Watercress
Wax gourd
Yardlong beans

*Spinach, Swiss chard, collard greens, kale and beet greens should only be eaten when cooked due to oxalate content when raw.

Starchy Vegetables[72]

Each of the following serving sizes contains approximately fifteen grams of carbohydrates.

Food Item	Serving Size
Acorn squash	½ cup
Artichoke	1 cup
Beets	1 cup
Burdock root	½ cup
Butternut squash	2/3 cup
Carrots	1 cup
Corn	½ cup
Green peas	½ cup
Jerusalem artichoke	½ cup
Jicama	2/3 cup
Lima beans	½ cup
Lotus root	½ cup
Okra	1 cup
Parsnip	2/3 cup
Potato (baked)	½ medium
Rutabaga	¼ large
Sweet potato or yam	½ medium
Turnip	½ cup

Legumes and Vegetables

Legumes are nutrient-rich and include many vitamins, minerals, phytonutrients (plant nutrients), antioxidants, dietary fiber, and protein. The dietary fiber helps digestion by slowing the rate at which food leaves the stomach, helping you to feel full after a meal and hopefully avoid that favorite pastime of pregnant ladies everywhere—snacking. Legumes are also high in starch, which breaks down to sugar during the digestion process. Because of the high starch content, they are also known to cause digestive issues, flatulence, an inflammatory response, and dysfunction in the gut. Soaking beans has been shown to reduce the sugar content, which causes these issues. Some raw beans contain potentially toxic substances that will diminish if soaked overnight before cooking. Of the beans listed below, the ones I recommend soaking are marked with asterisks. Be sure to discard the soaking water. Each of the following serving sizes contains approximately fifteen grams of carbohydrates.

Food Item	Serving Size
Black beans*	1/3 cup
Broad beans (fava beans)	1/3 cup
Chickpeas (garbanzo, Bengal)*	1/3 cup
Cowpeas (black-eyed peas)	½ cup
Cranberry beans	1/3 cup
French beans*	1/3 cup
Great Northern beans*	1/3 cup
Garbanzo beans*	1/3 cup
Hyacinth beans	1/3 cup
Kidney beans*	1/3 cup
Lentils	1/3 cup
Lupins	1 cup
Moth beans	1/3 cup
Mung beans	1/3 cup
Navy beans*	1/3 cup
Pigeon peas	1/3 cup
Pink beans*	1/3 cup
Pinto beans*	1/3 cup
Split peas	1/3 cup
White beans	1/3 cup
Yellow beans	1/3 cup

*Should be soaked overnight (eight hours). Will lessen cooking time and make bean easier to digest.

Daily recommendation:

- Legumes are considered a starchy vegetable and should make up no more than two servings per day of your total vegetable intake.
- If blood sugar issues are present, starchy vegetables should be reduced to three or four servings per week.

<u>Fruits</u>

Organic, fresh fruits are one of the richest sources of water-soluble vitamins when compared to all other food groups. We need to eat fruits every day because the human body needs a regular, ongoing supply of water-soluble vitamins since they cannot be stored in the body for future use like fat-soluble vitamins. The body also cannot produce them—they must come from the food we eat (called "essential vitamins").

Fruits are not all created equal, however. While all fruits are a concentrated source of carbohydrates and varying amounts of sugar, some are more sweet than others and will therefore have a greater adverse effect on blood sugar levels. Dried fruits are processed in a manner that removes many nutrients but increases sugar content, making them undesirable as a source of fruit, and as a result, they are not included in this list.

Maintaining stable blood glucose levels during pregnancy is critical to avoid gestational diabetes, which we covered earlier in this chapter. Most doctors watch for early warning signs of this condition so it can be addressed immediately when discovered. But you will be way ahead of the game by simply paying attention to how much sugar you have in your diet, which includes limiting the number of sugary fruits you consume. Fruits that are moderately high on the Glycemic Index are marked with an asterisk below. Fruits that are very high on the index are marked with two asterisks and should be avoided or consumed sparingly in small quantities.[73]

Daily recommendations:

- Fruits should make up no more than 10 percent of daily diet.
- Have one or two servings per day of low-glycemic fruits.
- Have one serving per day of moderate-glycemic fruit.
- High-glycemic fruits should be consumed in small quantities (¼ cup) and only on an occasional basis as a snack or dessert.

Each portion size is equal to approximately fifteen grams of carbohydrates.

Food Item	Serving Size
Acerola cherries	15
Apple—red*	1 small
Apple—green	1 small
Applesauce (unsweetened)*	½ cup
Apricots	2 medium
Avocado	1
Banana**	½ small
Blackberries	¾ cup
Blueberries	½ cup
Boysenberries	¾ cup

Breadfruit	⅛ small
Carambola	1 ½ cups
Cherries*	12
Crabapples	½ cup
Currants	1 cup
Dates**	2 medium
Elderberries	½ cup
Figs*	2 medium
Gooseberries	1 cup
Grapefruit	½ cup
Grapes**	15
Guavas	1 ½
Honeydew*	⅛ medium
Java-plum	¾ cup
Jujube	¼ cup
Kiwi*	1 large
Kumquats	5
Lemons	3 medium
Limes	2 medium
Litchis	7
Loganberries	¾ cup
Longans	31
Loquats	5 large
Mango	½ small
Melons (cantaloupe)	1 ½ cups
Melons (casaba)	1 ½ cups
Mulberries	1 cup
Nectarines*	1 small
Oranges*	1 small
Papaya*	1 cup
Passion fruit	3
Peach*	1 medium

Pear	½ large
Persimmon	½ medium
Pineapple*	¾ cup
Plantains	⅓ cup
Pomegranates	½
Plum*	2 medium
Prickly pears	1 ½ medium
Prunes**	3 medium
Quince	1 medium
Raisins**	2 tablespoons
Raspberries	1 cup
Rhubarb	7 stalks
Sapote	½ medium
Strawberries	1 ¼ cup
Sun-dried tomatoes	⅙ ounce
Tamarinds	15
Tangerines	2 small
Tomato	1 medium
Watermelon**	1 ¼ cups

Herbs and Spices

Herbs are generally considered safe and highly effective as remedies for common health complaints, as well as when used in small amounts when cooking food. Herbal beverages and nutritious teas are known to be safe during pregnancy when used in moderation, such as red raspberry, spearmint, chamomile, lemon balm, nettles, and rose hips.

I use herbs frequently in my private practice with clients, either individual herbs or blended formulas. But not all herbs are appropriate to use for daily or regular consumption during pregnancy, especially the first trimester. Some are known to carry risks during pregnancy and should be used only under the guidance of an herbalist. These are covered in more detail in Chapter 7.

Healthy Condiments

Condiments are considered a processed food and typically contain a variety of unwanted ingredients such as excess sugar (usually in the form of fructose), soy, preservatives, food dyes, sodium, food additives, and texture or taste enhancers such as monosodium glutamate (MSG).[74] Each of these ingredients carry with them potential health risks.[75] It's easy to assume they aren't harmful because we typically use only a small quantity of each one. Well, unless you eat like I used to—a little bit of hamburger with a pile of mayonnaise was a perfect lunch. Or how about smothering a baked potato with sour cream and bacon bits? Very yummy, but unfortunately those couple of teaspoons at each meal has a very negative, cumulative effect on the human body. The scariest part is a lot of these non-food ingredients are hormone disrupters.[76]

Alternatives to your typical condiment brands include searching out your own recipes for a homemade approach, or shopping for condiments where you will have healthy options to chose from. Check labels for organic ingredients, gluten-free, sugar-free, and soy-free choices.

Balsamic and other vinegars
Homemade sauces
Natural Mustard
Mayonnaise (no-sugar,
made with olive oil)

Olives
Salsa (without sugar)
Tamari (low-sodium soy sauce)

Summary of Dietary Recommendations during Pregnancy

Dairy
Daily and weekly recommendations:

- Dairy products are part of the protein food group.
- Dairy should be consumed in small quantities or eliminated.
- If choosing dairy, always purchase organic, antibiotic-free, hormone-free products from grass-fed livestock.
- For cow-milk substitutes, consider unsweetened hemp, almond, or coconut milks.

Omega-3 and -6 Fats
Daily and weekly recommendations:

- Consume 340 grams (two 6-ounce servings) per week of seafood or high-quality grass-fed beef.[77] (See food lists in Chapter 4.)
- Focus on a combination of omega-3 food sources and a high-quality fish-oil supplement to ensure you reach the proper amount of DHA fats, approximately 600 mg or more per day.[78]
- Limit seafood intake to wild-caught only to avoid exposure to mercury toxicity or other neurotoxins.[79] Avoid types of fish known to be high in mercury and other toxins (shellfish, shark, swordfish, king mackerel, tilefish, marlin, orange roughy, tuna).
- Consume high-quality, organic, grass-fed beef or bison up to three times per week.

- Include a high-quality EPA/DHA fish-oil supplement with your supplement regiment, minimum of 600 mg per day of DHA.
- Avoid using fats and oils with high omega-6 content. (See food lists in Chapter 4.)

Proteins
Daily Recommendations:

- Protein should make up approximately 25 percent of daily diet, or sixty to seventy-five grams of protein per day during first trimester.
- Protein sources should be varied and include organic eggs and high-quality, organic meats and fish (wild-caught).

Grains
Daily recommendations:

- Gluten-free grains only, should make up less than 1 percent of daily diet, or one small serving per day (examples: one slice of gluten-free bread, four or five crackers, half a cup of gluten-free pasta).
- Choose products that are made with gluten-free grains.
- If blood sugar issues are present or other health concerns, limit gluten-free grains to maximum of three times per week.

Vegetables
Daily recommendations:

- Starchy vegetables should make up no more than two servings per day of total vegetable intake, or no more than 5 percent of daily diet. If blood sugar issues are present, starchy vegetables should be reduced to a maximum of three or four servings per week.

- A vegetable is considered high in starch if it contains more than five grams of carbohydrates per half cup.
- Choose vegetables from organic sources.
- Consume legumes only after soaking and cooking.

Daily recommendations:

- Non-starchy vegetables should make up 60 percent of daily diet.
- Choose vegetables from organic sources.
- Eat a variety of vegetables.
- Consume at least five servings or two and one-half cups of non-starchy vegetables per day, a minimum of one with each meal.
- A portion of daily vegetable intake can be liquefied in a high-powered blender and consumed by drinking. See Appendix for vegetable juice recipe.
- Eat vegetables barely cooked (crunchy texture) as often as possible, except for spinach, Swiss chard, and beet greens, which should be thoroughly steamed or boiled to minimize the oxalate content.[80]

Fruits
Daily recommendations:

- Fruits should make up no more than 10 percent of daily diet.
- One or two servings per day of low-glycemic fruits

- One serving per day of moderate-glycemic fruit.
- High-glycemic fruits should be consumed in small quantities (one quarter cup) and only occasionally as a snack or dessert.

Summary of Foods to Avoid during Pregnancy

The following list of foods to avoid during pregnancy does not take into consideration other pre-existing health conditions that may require a stricter food-elimination plan.

Animal Protein to Avoid

- Bacon (except turkey bacon without nitrates and hormones—choose gluten-free)
- Hot dogs (except chicken and turkey hot dogs without nitrates and hormones—choose gluten-free)
- Tuna (all types—toro, albacore, ahi, including canned)

Grains to Avoid

- Barley
- Breads (unless gluten-free, sugar-free)
- Cereals (except gluten- and sugar-free varieties)
- Crackers (unless gluten- and sugar-free)
- Farro
- Kamut
- Oats (gluten-free okay)
- Pasta (unless made from brown rice, buckwheat, quinoa)
- Pastries
- Rye
- Spelt
- Triticale

- White flours
- White rice
- Wheat (refined)
- Whole wheat

Vegetables to Avoid

- Corn
- Mushrooms
- Potatoes (or eat sparingly, two or three servings per week)
- Beans and legumes (small amounts only, three or four servings per week, soak overnight before eating)

Nuts and Seeds to Avoid

- Cashews
- Peanuts, peanut butter

Oils to Avoid

- Canola oil
- Corn oil
- Cottonseed oil
- Peanut oil
- Processed oils and partially hydrogenated or fully hydrogenated oils
- Soy oil

Dairy to Avoid

- Cheeses (unless aged or organic. Eat in small quantities only, three or four servings per week.)

- Buttermilk
- Cow's milk
- Ice cream (infrequently for snacks only)
- Margarine
- Sour cream
- Yogurt (unless organic or from grass-fed sources. Choose brands with fewer than 10 g of sugar and consume infrequently, three or four servings per week)

*Note: pregnant and nursing women should not consume raw dairy products.

Fruits to Avoid

The following fruits are high on the glycemic index and are best to avoid, or should be consumed infrequently and in small quantities, two or three servings per week.

- Apricots
- Bananas
- Cherries
- Cranberries (sweetened)
- Dried fruits (including dates, figs, raisins, prunes)
- Guavas
- Grapes
- Juices (all, sweetened and unsweetened)
- Kiwis
- Mangoes
- Melons
- Nectarines
- Oranges
- Papyas

- Peaches
- Pears
- Pineapples
- Plums
- Persimmons
- Pomegranates
- Tangerines

Beverages to Avoid

- Alcohol
- Caffeinated teas (except green tea)
- Coffee (caffeinated and decaffeinated)
- Energy drinks (including vitamin waters)
- Fruit juices
- Kefir
- Kombucha
- Sodas (diet or regular)
- Rice and soy milks

Condiments to Avoid

Purchase condiments that are sugar-free, gluten-free, and organic whenever possible. Condiments should be used sparingly and infrequently.

- Gravy
- James and jellies
- Ketchup
- Mayonnaise
- Mustard
- Pickles

- Relish
- Salad dressings
- Sauces with vinegars and sugar
- Soy sauce and tamari sauce
- Spices that contain yeast, sugar, or other additives
- Vinegars (except raw, unfiltered apple cider vinegar, and unsweetened rice vinegar)
- Worcestershire sauce

Sweeteners

- Agave nectar
- Artificial sweeteners (aspartame, Nutrasweet, saccharin, acesulfame, and sucralose or Splenda)
- Barley malt
- Brown rice syrup
- Brown sugar
- Coconut sugar/nectar
- Corn syrup
- Dextrose Erythritol (Nectresse, Swerve, Truvia)
- Fructose (products sweetened with fruit juice)
- Honey (raw or processed)
- Maltitol
- Mannitol
- Maltodextrin
- Maple Syrup
- Molasses
- Raw or evaporated cane juice
- Sorbitol
- White sugar
- Yacon syrup

Miscellaneous to Avoid

- Cacao/chocolate (unless sweetened with stevia or xylitol)
- Candy
- Carob
- Cookies
- Donuts
- Fast food and fried foods
- Fermented foods (kimchi, sauerkraut, tempeh, yogurt, nutritional yeast, cultured vegetables, and so forth)
- Fruit strips
- Gelatin
- Gum
- Jerky (beef or turkey)
- Lozenges/mints
- Muffins
- Pastries
- Pizza
- Processed food
- Smoked, dried, pickled, and cured foods

Get Yourself Organized

When beginning a new dietary program or making a few changes to how you eat, when you eat, or adding supplements to your daily plan, organization is key to consistency. Here are a few tips that will help you stay on track.

- Create your own your personalized glycemic rating list of foods you like to eat. Keep it with you until you become familiar with it to help keep track of and monitor your sugar/carbohydrate intake.

- Have a copy of your daily supplement list with you or located in easily accessible locations in your home. For instance, I keep my list in my bathroom, where I take my morning and nighttime supplements, and a copy in my kitchen, where I take my meal-time supplements.
- Maintain a copy of your daily food groups and "foods to eat/foods to avoid" list. Keep it with you until you become very familiar with it, especially when eating out.
- If you are taking individual nutritional supplements in addition to or as a replacement for a prenatal multivitamin, consider using a daily pill box to organize supplements. I have two weeks of pill boxes that I pre-fill. They are convenient, travel-size pill boxes with four compartments for every day of the week. If you are leaving for the day, just grab the box for the day of the week, toss it in your purse or briefcase before heading out, and you have all your supplements for each meal. Of course, you still have to get in the habit of remembering to take them!

The Baby-Maker Strategy: Your Strategies for Fertility, Pre-Conception, and Pregnancy

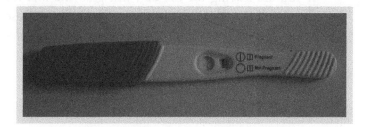

Source: Flickr.com. Used with permission.

*"A goal without
a plan is
just a wish."*

—*Antoine de Saint-Exupery*

146

In previous chapters, I talked to you about the importance of planning for pregnancy. Although it will seem to many of you that creating a health plan, timeline, and goals for having a baby diminishes the magic and wonder of it all, doing so is truly one of the most important steps you will take as future parents. The single, most impactful action you can take that will affect your child for its entire life is for you to be healthy when you conceive, as well as throughout your pregnancy. Think about it. What greater gift could you possibly give to your baby than to pass along a predisposition for good health and longevity?

Following the detailed recommendations and strategy that this chapter outlines is the key to your success. The pages that follow offer specific nutritional and lifestyle suggestions for pre-conception (one plan for women and another for men), pregnancy, supplement recommendations during pre-conception and pregnancy, as well as a chart of nutrients required during breastfeeding. With this information, balanced and healthful food choices (learned in Chapter 4), as well as recommendations on how to protect your microbiome (learned in Chapter 3), and lastly, important things to avoid (Chapter 7), you should be off to the baby races in no time!

Pre-Conception Strategy for Women

As you read through the list of key steps to optimize your health to improve fertility, one of the first questions that will pop into your mind is, *How long do I need to do this?* My hope is that you will be so amazed at how good you feel after just two to three weeks on this program that you won't be able to imagine going back to your old way of eating. Adopting these changes as permanent lifestyle modifications will be one of the best things you can do for your long-term health and future. You will dramatically increase your chances of avoiding major diseases and will add years to your lifespan.

Your start date for each of the steps outlined below, and beginning the supplement recommendations, should be six to eight months prior to your planned date for conception. If you are dealing with a chronic disease such as diabetes, chronic fatigue syndrome, or an autoimmune condition, it is possible that your body will need considerably longer. In these cases, working with a nutritionist or other healthcare practitioner is advised in order to properly address specific nutritional or health concerns.

To answer the earlier question about how long the average woman will need to follow this plan, I recommend these guidelines:

Women will switch over to the pregnancy strategy outlined below once your little bundle of joy is "in the oven," which will take you through pregnancy and delivery. There are additional guidelines and recommendations in Chapter 8 to help you with common issues following delivery and while breastfeeding. Continue with these recommendations until you stop breastfeeding or are one year from the date you delivered, whichever comes first. Always double-check any changes in diet, supplements and exercise with your doctor or healthcare practitioner before implementing them.

Changing how you eat might seem easy on the surface, but it's not. Most people find it surprisingly challenging. Your motivation to get pregnant is a driving force that will help keep you focused and determined. Remember: Your end goal is to deliver into your waiting arms the healthiest baby possible. This is hard work, but all for the sake of your health and the health of your unborn child. How's that for motivation!

Eleven Key Steps to Fertility—Women

Start Date: Six to Eight Months Prior to Conception

Step #1—Stop smoking, discontinue excessive alcohol consumption, and stop recreational drugs. This is critical so I am putting this first. Smoking, alcohol (excessive use), and drugs are poisonous substances to your body and will have damaging effects on your fertility, can stunt the growth of your fetus, and cause below average IQ development in your children. You cannot be an effective, engaged, responsible parent if you are abusing alcohol or drugs. If you are going to the trouble of analyzing and improving your diet to increase your odds of fertility and conception, then start by eliminating the things that are the most destructive habits. *These are show-stoppers.* Nicotine, drugs, and alcohol have no place in your life! **Goal:** *Immediately and permanently discontinue cigarette smoking, excessive alcohol consumption, and use of recreational drugs.*

Step #2—Discontinue use of oral contraceptives. Oral contraceptives rob the body of zinc and other nutrients that are critical to a fertile environment.

Goal: *Discontinue use of oral contraceptives.*

Step #3—Do a pre-conception detox. A cleansing fast helps flush out any toxins that have accumulated from a poor diet of processed, refined and sugary foods, use of recreational or pharmaceutical drugs, alcohol, environmental toxins, or exposure to viruses. Toxins have a detrimental effect on the fertility of sperm and eggs and can ultimately affect the health of the baby.[1] In the Appendix you will find a recipe for a detoxifying green drink, a delicious antioxidant salad, as well as more details on how and why to do a detoxification that includes a list of detoxifying foods and herbs.

Goal: *Do a five-to-seven–day cleansing fast or detoxification. See the Appendix for recipes and pre-conception detoxification information.*

Step #4—Eliminate inflammatory and toxic foods. Eliminate as many foods as possible that contain sugar, yeast, gluten, soy, and dairy, as well as foods that are processed or anything purchased from a fast-food restaurant. Processed foods are defined as foods that are packaged in boxes, cans, or bags. If it comes in a package of some sort and is not labeled "organic," then it will likely contain artificial ingredients, chemicals, preservatives, and other substances that are harmful to your health and your fertility.

Inflammatory foods and substances and foods that contain toxins have a way of clogging up our internal systems and preventing the healthy stuff from getting where it needs to go to do its job properly in the body. According to Trudy Scott, author of *The Antianxiety Food Solution*, celiac disease (an autoimmune disorder) or gluten sensitivity is a suspected cause of infertility in over 5 percent of women whose condition is otherwise unexplained.[2] Gluten is discussed in more detail in Chapter 4, and a list of food sources and other products that contain gluten can be found in the Appendix.

Most people have no idea how much of these substances is contained in the foods you eat on a daily basis. Even nutrition labels can be vague and difficult to decipher. Focus on the section labeled "other ingredients" on food labels. Work toward developing a habit of glancing at the label before dropping an item in your grocery cart. In order to eliminate harmful substances, it's important to become familiar with the ingredients typically found in your favorite foods.

Goal: *Foods in this category should be less than 20 percent of your daily food intake.*

Step #5—Eat organic foods. By eating organic foods, you are eliminating a vast array of toxins. Eat lots of organic eggs, quality organic butter from grass-fed cows, cream, fermented organic dairy products, and vegetables with special focus on leafy green veggies that are high in folic acid (folate), as well as legumes and seafood. (Avoid seafood that may contain mercury.) Include large amounts of organic organ meats if you have the palate for them. These would include tongue, kidneys, tripe, liver, and brain. Organ meats are extremely high in nutrients such as protein, iron, copper, folate, and vitamins A and B.

Goal: *80–90 percent of daily diet comes from organic sources.*

Step #6—Drink filtered or purified water. Most sources of drinking water contain unhealthy levels of toxins that, over time, bring danger to your quest for fertility. The list of chemicals typically identified in water includes arsenic, fluoride, and chlorine. It might surprise you to learn that the biggest culprit out of all of them is fluoride.[3] I know, I know—fluoride is supposed to be good for us, especially for our teeth, as evidenced by the fact that nearly every single brand of toothpaste proudly contains it (as does some bottled water, baby formulas and other products). But here are the facts:

The debates about fluoride have been going on for more than six decades. Numerous studies have confirmed it is a dangerous, toxic poison that accumulates in the body, and there is no data to support its effectiveness in the fight against tooth decay.[4] Furthermore, a 2009 study discovered that substances found in tap water were associated with thyroid disease, cancer, and immune-system deficiency and—you guessed it—"dramatically increased the odds of infertility anywhere from 70 to 154 percent."[5] So for the sake of your fertility, please, no more tap water!

Goal: Drink half your body weight in ounces daily of purified or filtered water (e.g. 120 pound woman should drink 60 ounces of water per day). Do not count alcoholic beverages, soda, coffee, or flavored water.

Step #7—Keep stress at a minimum. Stress activates the fight-or-flight response from the adrenal glands, which impact hormone regulation big time. If your hormones are out of whack, you are much more likely to have problems with fertility and conception.[6] You don't need to become a master yogi to keep your adrenal glands from working overtime. A short ten-minute session of meditation or deep breathing is enough to restore balance and calm the chemical cascade that begins when a stress response is activated. If ongoing stress is a major issue for you, it may be worthwhile to consider counseling, hypnosis, or some other more intensive therapy to reduce your body's response to the stressor.

Goal: Stress-reducing activity ten minutes per day, five to seven days per week.

Step #8—Start taking a prenatal vitamin or other high-potency multivitamin. Compare the ingredients in your prenatal vitamin or multivitamin to the other nutrient dosages recommended in this book. Add separate, individual nutrients if your prenatal or multi are not at the recommended levels. Important note: Do *not* exceed the recommended dosages. When taking supplements, more is *not* better. If you believe you need a higher dose of a particular nutrient than what is recommended here, check with your obstetrician, medical doctor, or other healthcare practitioner before increasing.

Step #9—Take additional supplements every day.

- Folate or 5-MTHF—Studies show that folate plays a vital role in female reproduction, oocyte (immature egg cell in ovary) quality and maturation, implantation, placentation, fetal growth, and organ development.[7] An artificial form of folate is often used in supplements called "folic acid." It is best to use folate (from food sources) or 5-MTHF (the activated form), which are more effective, more highly absorbable sources of this nutrient and can help improve fertility. Check to see whether folate or MTHF is an ingredient in your prenatal vitamin or multivitamin. If it is, there is no need to take it as a separate supplement.

Dosage: 800 mcg per day.

- Fish oil, EPA + DHA—Essential fatty acids, including cod liver oil, are excellent sources of omega-3 fatty acids that support fertility. They are also easy to get from foods, so I have included a list of foods that are high in omega-3 fatty acids in Chapter 4. For the purposes of improving fertility, however, adding a fish-oil supplement will ensure you are receiving an optimal dose and improve the balance of omega 3s to 6s. (The body needs both.) DHA is the more important one for pregnancy. A dose of at least 600 mg of DHA per day is recommended. See Chapter 4, the section on Foods That Contain Omega-3 Fatty Acids.

Dosage: *2,000 mg per day, minimum of 600 mg of, which should be DHA.*

- Probiotic—probiotics help normalize and support the level of healthy bacteria in the gut as well as the vaginal microbiome environment in your body. Both are important to your overall health when planning for conception. A combination of probiotic strains is needed since the gut is colonized with multiple bacterial strains, whereas the vagina contains predominantly Lactobacillus.

Dosage: *Five to ten billion organisms per day, combination of probiotic strains.*

- Antioxidant—Antioxidants help restore balance to our internal detoxification processes. When you hear the term "oxidative stress," it refers to a condition when these processes are out of balance. If left unchecked, oxidative stress can contribute to a long list of health concerns, including infertility. To better understand all of this, think about how iron looks when it is rusting. The rusting is caused by oxidation, which is a term for a molecular change to other molecules that is very damaging, and it occurs in the human body probably more often than it occurs on our cars and bicycles. In addition to causing damage to cells and tissues, oxidation also produces dangerous and harmful byproducts, which contribute to the total burden called "oxidative stress." Along with oxidation, the body's internal detoxification processes must contend with assaults from other things like toxins in the air, processed food, poor-quality water, excessive alcohol consumption, and smoking.

Research has shown that oxidative stress in women can delay the ability to conceive, decrease fertilization rates, decrease egg viability, and lower implantation rates.[8] Taking an antioxidant as part of your pre-conception plan will help reduce free radicals and support the normal detoxification process that occurs in the body. There are many to choose from. Pine Bark Extract (100–300 mg per day), Resveratrol (100–300 mg per day), CoQ10 (100–200 mg per day), or a blended formula such as Pure Encapsulations Antioxidant Formula would all be effective.

Dosage: *Choose a single antioxidant or blended formula. Follow manufacturer's instructions.*

- Vitamin D3 + Vitamin K2—Ask your healthcare provider to order a blood test to check your vitamin D level (test is called 25 (OH)D). Vitamin D deficiency is currently at epidemic proportions in the U.S. and worldwide and is directly linked to infertility in men and women. The recommended level for adults is 50–70 ng/ml.[9] If your levels are below that or at the bare minimum (<50 ng/ml) and you rarely get sun exposure, adding a vitamin D3 supplement to your plan is essential. Vitamin K2 (MK-7 form) helps to shuttle calcium directly into the bones should be taken along with D3. Dosage: 5,000 to 8,000 IU per day (to elevate levels above 40 ng/ml) + 50–100 mcg of K2.

- Iron—iron deficiency is the most common nutritional deficiency in women and can cause infertility. Adequate formation of red blood cells, DNA formation, transport of oxygen to tissues, as well as other functions are all dependent on proper levels of iron within the body. According to the Nurses' Health Study II, women who consumed iron supplements had a 60 percent lower risk of infertility than women who did not.[10] Typically, a prenatal vitamin will contain a sufficient dosage of iron, but if you are anemic or your iron level tested low, then an additional supplement of iron is required. Be aware that the substantial need for iron during conception and pregnancy cannot be met through diet alone. Also pay attention to what type of iron is included in a supplement. Ferrous sulfate iron is known to cause constipation or gastrointestinal issues. Ferrous succinate, ferrous glycinate, ferrous fumarate, or ferrous pyrophosphate are the most bioavailable and cause the fewest side effects. Pure Essence has a retail product called Blood Builder, which is 26 mg of iron primarily from food sources. It is known to be easy on the gut and not cause constipation.

Dosage: *30 mg, twice per day or follow manufacturer's instructions.*

Important note: Not all supplements are created equal. For additional information on how and where to purchase supplements, please refer to Chapter 9.

Step #10—Get plenty of sleep and exercise. Regular, adequate sleep and exercise are nourishing and restorative for the body. Exercise helps keep fluids moving, stimulates the immune system and digestive and detoxification systems, and ensures production of much-needed enzymes and hormones. Don't overdo your workouts, though. Studies have revealed that women of average weight who engaged in vigorous exercise like running, swimming, and aerobics for five or more hours a week were *42 percent less likely to get pregnant* than women who did not exercise at all.[11] A good night's sleep provides significant benefits and provides critical support to the immune system, metabolism, cognitive functions, and detoxification. Studies indicate that the average amount of sleep needed to reap these benefits for an adult is seven to nine hours each night.

Goal: *Seven to nine hours of continuous sleep every night and twenty to thirty minutes of moderate exercise three or four times per week.*

Step #11—Cut back on caffeine. A lot of us like our caffeine in the morning, often followed up later in the day by a super-sized soda, but if you're trying to get pregnant, you need to reconsider both. A study published in the *British Journal of Pharmacology* in 2011 revealed findings that two cups of coffee reduced the muscle activity in the fallopian tubes to the point where they couldn't do their job of transporting the woman's eggs from her ovaries to the womb.[12]

Goal: *Maximum of one cup per day of light to moderate brewed coffee.*

For details on foods to eat and foods to be avoided, please refer to Chapter 4 and the Summary of Foods to Avoid list in the Appendix.

Pre-Conception Strategy for Men—
Ten Key Steps for Fertility

<u>Start Date: Six to Eight Months Prior to Conception</u>

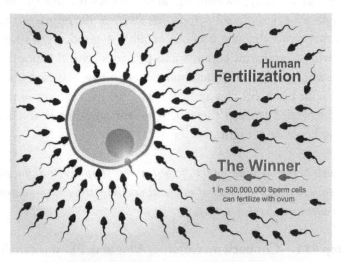

Source: BigstockPhoto.com. Used with permission.

Men's health is as vital to a couple's ability to conceive as the woman's. We all instinctively believe our virile, strong, loving men have virile, strong, highly capable little swimmers, but that isn't always the case.

Since the woman, by far, bears the biggest burden of a pregnancy, (and many would argue through child-rearing as well), this is a perfect opportunity for all future dads to step up to the plate. What better time than right now to demonstrate your commitment as a caring, concerned, engaged partner and parent by getting yourself healthy inside and out?

The strategy timeline for men begins around the same time as women: six to eight months prior to the date of your planned conception. If you are dealing with a chronic disease such as diabetes, chronic fatigue syndrome, or an autoimmune condition, it is possible that your body will need considerably longer. In these cases, working with a nutritionist or other healthcare practitioner is advised in order to properly address specific nutritional or health concerns.

How long you should continue with your dietary plan is obviously very different for men than for women. Once your "boys" have done their job and your stew is in the pot, so to speak, technically you can resume your old diet. As I mentioned above for women, for the sake of your long-term health and longevity, I hope you continue on a modified, holistic, whole-foods diet for years to come.

Step #1—Stop smoking, discontinue excessive alcohol consumption, and stop recreational drugs. This is so important and bears repeating from the section above for women. Smoking, alcohol use (excessive), and drugs are poisonous substances to your body and will have damaging effects on your fertility, can stunt the growth of the fetus, and cause below-average IQ development in your children.[13] You cannot be an effective, engaged, responsible parent if you are abusing alcohol or drugs. Let me be blunt: There is no point eliminating the junk food or taking the other health-restoring measures listed here if you aren't taking your health and fertility seriously enough to discontinue smoking, excessive alcohol consumption, and/or drugs. *These are show-stoppers.* Your inability or unwillingness to take this step should have you questioning your commitment to conceive and raise a child.

Goal: *Immediately and permanently discontinue cigarette smoking, excessive alcohol consumption, and use of recreational drugs.*

Step #2—Do a pre-conception detox. A cleansing fast helps flush out any toxins that have accumulated from a poor diet of processed, refined, and sugary foods, use of recreational or pharmaceutical drugs, alcohol consumption, environmental toxins, or exposure to viruses. Toxins have a very detrimental effect on the fertility of sperm in men, just as they do on the eggs in women.[14] In the Appendix you will find a recipe for a detoxifying green drink, a delicious antioxidant salad, as well as more details on how and why to do a detoxification that includes a list of detoxifying foods and herbs.

Goal: *Do a five-to-seven–day cleansing fast or bowel or colon detoxification. See section on recipes for suggestions on cleansing and detoxifying foods.*

Step #3—Eliminate inflammatory and toxic foods. Eliminate as many foods as possible that contain sugar, yeast, gluten, soy, and dairy, as well as foods that are processed or anything purchased from a fast-food restaurant. Processed foods are defined as foods that are packaged in boxes, cans or bags. If it comes in a package of some sort and is not labeled "organic," then it will likely contain artificial ingredients, chemicals, preservatives, and other substances that are harmful to your health and your fertility.[15]

Goal: Keep foods in this category to less than 20 percent of your daily food intake or no more than two servings per day.

Step #4—Keep Stress at a minimum. Science hasn't exactly figured out why stress affects male fertility, but they know it does. For instance, we know that men who are under work-related stress can have diminished testosterone levels. Men who are unemployed will have greater chance of lower sperm quality than employed men. There's little doubt that ongoing stress in men is harmful to sperm and semen quality, affecting sperm concentration and ability to fertilize an egg.[16]

The biological reality is that it is very difficult to control or suppress the stress response, no matter whether you are a man or a woman. The stress response, or "fight or flight" is a normal, healthy response from the body that is meant to protect us. The threat to our fertility increases when stress is regularly activated or becomes chronic. Most people are not in a situation where they can quit a job for the sake of their stress levels. But you can look at other things to help your body better manage the stress response. So, men, find a healthy, wholesome activity that calms you and try to incorporate it into your daily routine for ten minutes a day. You don't need to become a master yogi or twist yourself into a Pilates pretzel to lower stress levels. Deep breathing, massage therapy, counseling, or even a slow, relaxing walk done on a regular basis will do the trick.

Goal: *Stress-reducing activity ten minutes per day, five to seven days per week.*

Step #5—Eat primarily organic foods. By eating organic foods, you are eliminating toxins that have negative effects on sperm performance. Eat lots of organic eggs, quality organic butter from grass-fed cows, cream, nuts and seeds, vegetables with special focus on leafy green veggies, as well as legumes and seafood. (Avoid seafood that may contain mercury.) Include large amounts of organic organ meats if you have the palate for them. These would include tongue, kidneys, tripe, liver, and brain. Organ meats are extremely high in nutrients such as protein, iron, copper, folate and vitamins A and B.

Goal: *80–90 percent of daily diet comes from organic sources.*

Step #6—Drink filtered or purified water. Most sources of drinking water contain unhealthy levels of toxins that, over time, bring danger to your sperm count, quality, and motility. The list of chemicals typically identified in water includes arsenic, fluoride, and chlorine, with fluoride being by far the most pervasive and dangerous to your health.

Goal: *Drink half your body weight in ounces daily of purified or filtered water. (e.g. a 180 pound man should drink about 90 ounces of water per day) Do not count alcoholic beverages, soda, coffee, or flavored water.*

Step #7—Take supplements every day.

- Vitamin C—improves semen quality, reduces oxidative stress.
  - Dosage: 1000 mg per day.
- Vitamin E—main antioxidant in sperm cell membranes.
  - Dosage: 400 IU per day.
- Vitamin A or Lycopene—antioxidant required for cell growth and health of testes and sperm.
  - Dosage:15,000 IU vitamin A or 5 mg Lycopene daily.
- Vitamin D3 and K2—Studies performed by fertility experts in Australian in 2008 found that almost a third of eight hundred infertile men had lower-than-normal levels of vitamin D3, making this vitamin a major culprit in contributing to infertility. One hundred of those men agreed to make and maintain lifestyle changes (Stop smoking, minimize caffeine and alcohol intake, lose weight, and so forth.) for three months prior to conception, along with a regimen of vitamins and antioxidants, including vitamin D. Eleven of them went on to achieve pregnancy naturally without IVF treatment.[17] Another study in 2009 confirmed that human sperm has a vitamin D receptor, meaning that it is very likely to play an important role in cell signaling in the male reproductive system. Ask your healthcare provider to order a blood test to check your vitamin D level. (The test is called 25 (OH)D.) Vitamin K2 (MK-7 form) should be taken along with D3 to help shuttle calcium into the bones. Dosage: 5,000 to 8,000 IU

per day of D3 (to elevate levels above 40 ng/ml) + 50–100 mcg of K2.

- Zinc—deficiencies in zinc will cause low testosterone which will affect sperm count. Important nutrient for healthy, fertile sperm.

Dosage: 30 mg per day.

- Selenium—antioxidant required for male fertility, normal sperm maturation, and motility.

Dosage: 200 mcg per day.

- Folate and Vitamin B12—both are concentrated in the head of sperm and required to protect DNA. B12 helps with sperm count and motility.

Dosage: 800 mcg per day each.

- Alpha-Lipoic Acid (ALA)—antioxidant that protects sperm, regenerates other antioxidants.

Dosage: 100 mg per day.

- Carnitine—provides protective antioxidant effects and energy to the testicles and sperm. Low levels of carnitine may be a contributing factor to male infertility.

Dosage: Up to 3000 mg per day for four months prior to conception.

- CoQ10—considered one of the most important antioxidants in sperm. It reduces oxidative stress in the head of the sperm and also enhances sperm motility and overall stamina thereby enhancing chances for conception.

Dosage: 200 mg per day.

(Murray and Pizzorno, revised 2012)[18]

Not all supplements are created equal. For additional information on how and where to purchase supplements, please refer to Chapter 9.

Step #8—Get plenty of sleep and exercise. Regular, adequate sleep and exercise is nourishing and restorative for a man's body, just as it is for a woman. Exercise helps keep fluids moving, stimulates the immune, digestive and detoxification systems, and ensures production of much needed enzymes and hormones. Also, similar to women, men do not want to go crazy with an intense exercise routine. Sperm quality responds best to a moderately intense exercise program that is done with consistency, rather than a high-intensity workout.[19] An example would be continuous running or jogging at a moderate speed for about thirty to forty minutes. Keep in mind, men, studies show that sperm count, shape, and quantity all dropped back to "normal" levels within a week after exercise stops.[20] Sperm motility hangs in there a little longer—your "guys" keep swimming better for about a month after you stop exercising.[21]

A good night's sleep provides significant benefits and provides critical support to the immune system, metabolism, cognitive functions and detoxification. Studies indicate that the average amount of sleep needed to reap these benefits for an adult is seven to nine hours each night.

Goal: Seven to nine hours of continuous sleep every night and thirty to forty minutes of moderate exercise four or five times per week.

Step #9—Cut back on caffeine. If you occasionally have caffeine (coffee, tea, chocolate) or keep it at a minimum (maximum of two cups of coffee per day), you are probably not consuming enough to cause fertility problems. However, excessive amounts of caffeine are known to cause issues with sperm motility. If you and your partner are having issues getting pregnant, caffeine should definitely be reduced or eliminated.[22]

Goal: Maximum of two cups per day of light to moderate brewed coffee.

Step #10 – Reduce your body's exposure to electromagnetics. Many studies are being done on the effects of radiofrequency electromagnetic waves on human semen. The waves emitted from cell phones (in talk mode and when the phone is often kept in a front trouser pocket), may drastically lower sperm production and impair male fertility.[23]

Goal: Do not carry a cell phone in a front trouser pocket.

Nutrition and Lifestyle Strategy during Pregnancy

Ladies, if you followed the Baby Maker—Eleven Key Steps for Fertility prior to conceiving, it's time to take inventory of what you are doing and not doing with your lifestyle and nutrition now that you are pregnant. Below is a repeat of several steps from the fertility and pre-conception strategy that you will want to follow throughout your extraordinary nine months of pregnancy.

1. No smoking, alcohol consumption, or recreational drugs.
2. Do not attempt to detoxify when pregnant. Do not consume detoxification teas or use fasting protocols or cleansing systems or products.
3. Continue avoiding inflammatory and toxic foods—foods containing sugar, yeast, gluten, soy, dairy, processed foods, fast foods.
4. Eat organic. Strive for getting 80–90 percent of your daily food intake from organic sources.
5. Drink half your body weight in ounces of filtered or purified water every day. (e.g. 140 pounds = approximately 70 ounces of water every day)
6. Keep stress at a minimum. Use stress-reducing activities if necessary, five to seven days per week for around ten minutes each day. Consider deep breathing, yoga, hypnosis, massage, meditation, or other therapies that work for you.
7. Start taking a prenatal vitamin or other high-potency multivitamin if you have not done so prior to conception. (See Supplement Recommendations for Pregnancy later in this chapter.)
8. Take additional supplements to augment your prenatal if specific nutrients are deficient when compared to the supplement recommendations listed. Please see the section on Supplement Recommendations for Pre-Conception and Pregnancy in this chapter. Also in this chapter you will find a list of my rec-

ommendations for prenatal multivitamins that are on the market for retail purchase. In most cases, you will definitely need a separate EPA + DHA fish oil that contains a minimum of 600 mg of DHA. Fish-oil requirements are rarely sufficient in pre-natal vitamins currently on the market, so an individual supplement is required in addition to food sources being consumed.

9. Get plenty of sleep and exercise. Regular, adequate sleep and light exercise is nourishing, restorative, and helps support the immune and digestive systems. For a restorative sleep cycle, pregnant women should be getting between seven and nine hours per night. Women who engaged in regular, strenuous exercise or sports activities prior to conception should always check with their healthcare provider for their recommendation on continuing them during pregnancy. In most cases, if it is something you have done consistently prior to pregnancy and your body is accustomed to it, you should be able to safely continue it.

10. Keep coffee and other caffeinated beverages to no more than one cup per day during pregnancy. (Best to eliminate caffeine completely.)

Summary of Dietary Recommendations during Pregnancy

The following recommendations are repeated below from Chapter 4. If you would like more information as to why a particular food is recommended or not during pregnancy, please refer back to Chapter 4 for these details and an explanation.

Dairy
Daily and Weekly Recommendations:

- Dairy products are part of the protein food group.
- Dairy should be consumed in small quantities or eliminated completely.
- If choosing dairy products, always purchase organic, antibiotic-free and hormone-free, and from grass-fed livestock.
- For cow-milk substitutes, consider unsweetened hemp, almond, or coconut milks.

Omega 3 and 6 Fats
Daily and Weekly Recommendations:

- Consume 340 grams (two 6-ounce servings) per week of seafood or high quality, grass-fed beef.[24] (See food lists in Chapter 4.)
- Focus on a combination of omega-3 food sources and a high quality fish-oil supplement to ensure you reach the proper amount of DHA fats, approximately 600 mg or more per day.[25]
- Important to limit seafood intake to wild-caught only to avoid exposure to mercury or other neurotoxins.[26] Avoid types of fish known to be high in mercury and other toxins (shellfish, shark, swordfish, king mackerel, tilefish, marlin, orange roughy, tuna).
- Consume high-quality, organic, grass-fed beef or bison up to three times per week.
- Include a high-quality EPA/DHA fish-oil supplement with your supplement regiment, minimum of 600 mg per day of DHA.

- Avoid using fats and oils with high omega-6 content. (See food lists in Chapter 4.)

Proteins
Daily Recommendations:

- Protein should make up approximately 25 percent of daily diet, or sixty to seventy-five grams of protein per day during first trimester.
- Protein sources should be varied and include organic eggs and high quality, organic meats and fish (wild-caught).

Grains
Daily Recommendations:

- Gluten-free grains only should make up less than 1 percent of daily diet, or one small serving per day (examples: one slice of gluten-free bread, four or five crackers, half a cup of gluten-free pasta).
- Choose products that are made with gluten-free grains.
- If blood sugar issues are present or other health concerns, limit gluten-free grains to maximum of three times per week.

Vegetables
Daily Recommendations:

- Starchy vegetables should make up no more than two servings per day of total vegetable intake, or no more than 5 percent of daily diet. If blood sugar issues are present, starchy vegetables should be reduced to three or four servings per week.

- A vegetable is considered high in starch if it contains more than 5 grams of carbohydrates per half-cup.
- Choose vegetables from organic sources
- Consume legumes only after soaking and cooking.
- *Daily Recommendations:*
- Non-starchy vegetables should make up approximately 60 percent of daily diet.
- Choose vegetables from organic sources
- Eat a variety of vegetables.
- Consume at least 5 servings or 2½ cups of non-starchy vegetables per day, a minimum of one with each meal.
- A portion of daily vegetable intake can be liquefied in a high-powered blender and consumed by drinking. (See Appendix for vegetable juice recipe.)
- Eat vegetables barely cooked (crunchy texture) as often as possible, except for spinach , Swiss chard and beet greens, which should be thoroughly steamed or boiled to minimize oxalate content.[27]

Fruits
Daily Recommendations:

- Fruits should make up no more than 10 percent of daily diet.
- 1 to 2 servings per day of low-glycemic fruits
- 1 serving per day of moderate-glycemic fruit
- High-glycemic fruits should be consumed in small quantities (¼ cup) and only on an occasional basis as a snack or dessert.

Summary of Foods to Avoid during Pregnancy

The following list of foods to avoid during pregnancy does not take into consideration other pre-existing health conditions that may require a stricter food elimination plan.

<u>Animal Protein to Avoid</u>

- Bacon (except turkey bacon without nitrates and hormones; choose gluten-free)
- Hot dogs (except chicken and turkey hot dogs without nitrates and hormones; choose gluten-free)
- Tuna (all types—toro, albacore, ahi and so forth, including canned)

<u>Grains to Avoid</u>

- Barley
- Breads (unless gluten-free, sugar-free)
- Cereals (except gluten- and sugar-free varieties)
- Crackers (unless gluten- and sugar-free)
- Farro
- Kamut
- Oats (gluten-free okay)
- Pasta (unless made from brown rice, buckwheat, quinoa)
- Pastries
- Rye
- Spelt
- Triticale
- White flours
- White rice

- Wheat (refined)
- Whole wheat

Vegetables to Avoid

- Corn
- Mushrooms
- Potatoes (or eat sparingly, two or three times per week)
- Beans and legumes (small amounts only, three or four times per week, soak overnight before eating)

Nuts and Seeds to Avoid

- Cashews
- Peanuts, peanut butter

Oils to Avoid

- Canola oil
- Corn oil
- Cottonseed oil
- Peanut oil
- Processed oils and partially hydrogenated or fully hydrogenated oils
- Soy oil

Dairy to Avoid*

- Cheeses (unless aged or organic, eat in small quantities only, three or four times per week)
- Buttermilk
- Cow's milk

- Ice cream (infrequently for snacks, small quantities only)
- Margarine
- Sour cream
- Yogurt (unless organic or from grass-fed sources, choose brands with less than 10 g of sugar, consume infrequently, three or four times per week)

*Note: pregnant and nursing women should not consume raw dairy products. It is also advised that consumption of all dairy products be reduced or eliminated during pregnancy.

Fruits to Avoid

The following fruits are high on the glycemic index and should be eliminated, or consumed infrequently and in small quantities, two or three times per week.

- Apricots
- Bananas
- Cherries
- Cranberries (sweetened)
- Dried Fruits (including dates, figs, raisins, prunes)
- Guavas
- Grapes
- Juices (all, sweetened and unsweetened)
- Kiwis
- Mangoes
- Melons
- Nectarines
- Oranges
- Papayas
- Peaches

- Pears
- Pineapples
- Plums
- Persimmons
- Pomegranates
- Tangerines

Beverages to Avoid

- Alcohol
- Caffeinated teas (except green tea)
- Coffee (caffeinated and decaffeinated)
- Energy drinks (including vitamin waters)
- Fruit juices
- Kefir
- Kombucha
- Sodas (diet or regular)
- Rice and soy milks

Condiments to Avoid

Purchase condiments that are sugar-free, gluten-free, and organic whenever possible. Condiments should be used sparingly and infrequently.

- Gravy
- James and jellies
- Ketchup
- Mayonnaise
- Mustard
- Pickles
- Relish

- Salad dressings
- Sauces with vinegars and sugar
- Soy sauce and tamari sauce
- Spices that contain yeast, sugar or other additives
- Vinegars (except raw, unfiltered apple cider vinegar and unsweetened rice vinegar)
- Worcestershire sauce

Sweeteners to Avoid

- Agave nectar
- Artificial sweeteners (aspartame, Nutrasweet, saccharin, acesulfame and sucralose or Splenda)
- Barley malt
- Brown rice syrup
- Brown sugar
- Coconut sugar/nectar
- Corn syrup
- Dextrose Erythritol (Nectresse, Swerve, Truvia)
- Fructose (products sweetened with fruit juice)
- Honey (raw or processed)
- Maltitol
- Mannitol
- Maltodextrin
- Maple Syrup
- Molasses
- Raw or evaporated cane juice
- Sorbitol
- White sugar
- Yacon syrup

<u>Miscellaneous to Avoid</u>

- Cacao/chocolate (unless sweetened with stevia or xylitol)
- Candy
- Carob
- Cookies
- Donuts
- Fast food and fried foods
- Fermented foods (kimchi, sauerkraut, tempeh, yogurt, nutritional yeast, cultured vegetables, and so forth)
- Fruit strips
- Gelatin
- Gum
- Jerky (beef or turkey)
- Lozenges/mints
- Muffins
- Pastries
- Pizza
- Processed food
- Smoked, dried, pickled, and cured foods

Supplement Recommendations for Pre-Conception and Pregnancy

After reviewing the list of supplement recommendations, please be sure to refer to Chapter 9, which will give you an understanding of not only which supplements to take, but also how to differentiate a good supplement from a poorly manufactured one. You are investing a lot of time and money to become educated and informed, all for the benefit of the beautiful little soul that is waiting for you. No point in cutting corners now!

Most prenatal multivitamin formulas will have varying amounts of the nutrients listed in the chart below. I have yet to find a prenatal formula that contains sufficient quantities of the most important of these, which means you will need to compare the dosage listed on your multi-prenatal formula and augment with individual supplements where it is deficient.

Be aware that in some multi-prenatal formulas you may notice many other nutrients as well, such as manganese, niacin, vitamin K, copper, or iodine. Although usually included in very small amounts (dosage), they are often included for their influence on absorption and effectiveness. Your focus should be on the "must-have"s listed below.

Must-Have Nutrients to Support Pregnancy

Supplement	Reason	Recommended Dose
Calcium + vitamin K2 (calcium preferably from algae)	• Calcium needs increase by 50 percent during pregnancy • Vitamin K2 shuttles calcium to bones and teeth • Supports development of fetus' bone structure • Keeps mother's bones and teeth strong	Cal.1000 mg/day—1st trimester K2 200–300 mcg Cal.1200 mg/day—2nd trimester K2 200–300 mcg Cal.1600 mg/day—3rd trimester K2 200–300 mcg

Iron (supplement with iron during 1st trimester only if blood tests show deficiency)	• Important if mother has tendency toward anemia • Helps improve fertility • Supports production of new cells	50–70 mg/day—2nd and 3rd trimesters (Look for Blood Builder by Pure Essence, 26 mg of iron from food sources primarily, easy on the gut, minimal if any constipation)
DHA fish oil (can be combination DHA/EPA, algae-derived is an excellent form of fish oil)	• Supports development of baby's nervous system, brain, eyes and heart • Helps prevent blood clotting • Prevents low birth weight • Decreases risk of premature birth	Min. 300 mg/day DHA—1st trimester Min. 600 mg/day DHA—by mid-2nd trimester Min. 600 mg/day DHA—3rd trimester
Folate or 5-MTHF (activated form of folic acid)	• Helps prevent neural tube defects • Stimulates mother's appetite during 1st trimester when morning sickness is common	800 mcg/day
Vitamin E	• Protective antioxidant support	400 IU/day
Vitamin A (use retinol form of vitamin A)	• Essential at time of conception for embryo development • Needed for healthy eyes, prevention of eye defects	2500 IU/day (5000 IU/day may be warranted if diet is deficient in vitamin A food sources)

Vitamin B12	• Important for cell reproduction and growth	500 mcg/day
Vitamin D3	• Important for baby's bone and hormone development • Supports mother's immune system	5000 IU/day
Probiotic (predominantly lactobacillus species)	• Build up good lactobacillus bacteria that is passed onto baby • Lessens risk of ear infections and illness in baby during first few years • Helps with constipation and supports mother's immune system	1 tablet/day take before bedtime (15–30 billion organisms)
Zinc	• Helps mother hold needed hormones to support pregnancy • Supports cell growth and division	30 mg/day
Selenium	• Helps prevent birth defects and miscarriages • Antioxidant protects against free radicals	200 mcg/day

Suggestions for Multivitamin Supplement Brands for Optimal Fertility, Pre-Conception, Prenatal

At the time of print, the supplements below were all widely available to you as a retail customer online and in holistic health food markets. As a reminder, depending on your diet and the nutrient values found in the multivitamin you choose, you will need to augment the multi- with individual nutrients/supplements to meet the minimum requirements for the stage you are at in your pregnancy.

- Jarrow Preg-Natal
- Garden of Life Organic Whole Food Prenatal Multi
- Vitanica Femecology Probiotic (for vaginal pH and microflora)
- Emerald Prenatal by Ultra Laboratories
- EPA/DHA Fish Oil—Ultra Pure Omega3 (available only through www.intelligentlabs.org) OR Wiley's Wild Alaskan Prenatal Fish Oil

Nutrient Requirements during Breastfeeding[28]

The following chart provides nutrient levels required during breastfeeding. Use it as a guideline when shopping for a multi- or post-natal vitamin. To reach the optimum nutrient levels, you may have to purchase individual nutritional supplements to augment the levels in your multi and get you where you need to be.

You will also find this chart in Chapter 8 as part of the section on nutrition during breastfeeding. In Chapter 8 the chart is accompanied by nutritional guidelines and corresponding food sources for each nutrient.

Nutrient	Daily Amount (minimum to safe maximum)
Calories	2,500–3,200
Fiber	25–45 g
Protein	65–90 g
Fluids	Approximately 3 quarts or 96 ounces.
Fish oil—omega 3-fatty acids (DHA + EPA)	Min. 300–600 mg
Vitamin A	7,000–10,000 IU
Vitamin D	400–600 IU
Vitamin K2	200–300 mcg/day
Vitamin E	400 IU
Vitamin B1 (Thiamin)	1.6–25.0 mg
Vitamin B2 (Riboflavin)	1.7–25.0 mg
Vitamin B3 (Niacin)	18–100 mg
Vitamin B5 (Pantothenic acid)	7–250 mg
Vitamin B6 (Pyridoxine)	2.5–100 mg
Vitamin B12 (Cobalamin)	4–200 mcg
Vitamin B9 (Folate or 5-MTHFR)	600–800 mcg
Biotin	200–500 mcg
Choline	100–250 mg
Inositol	100–250 mg
Vitamin C	120–2,000 mg
Bioflavonoids	125–250 mg
Calcium	1,200–1,600 mg
Chloride	2–4 g
Chromium	50–400 mcg
Copper	2–3 mg
Iodine	290–400 mcg

Iron	30–50 mg
Magnesium	450–1,000 mg
Manganese	2.5–15 mg
Molybdenum	150–250 mcg
Phosphorus	1,200–1,600 mg
Potassium	2–5 g
Selenium	150–300 mcg
Zinc	25–40 mg

You are now armed with a plan to improve your fertility, support and improve your health during pregnancy, and support your health during breastfeeding. Congratulations on your commitment to good health for you and your future child!

Now before you run off to load up on all that nourishing food, be sure to read through the other chapters in this book. They each contain information vital to successful implementation of your plan, and will further increase your chances of success.

Through my years of experience in private consultations with clients, I have also learned that there is more "buy-in" with major dietary changes when people understand the "why." You already know why you're doing this—in order to have a healthy conception and pregnancy. Why nutrition works is equally important, and that's what you will get from other sections of this book. So, for those of you who may have sneaked right over to this chapter to review "the plan," please be sure to spend some time reviewing the information contained in the other chapters. Your "why" depends on it!

Eating the Baby-Maker Way by Trimester: What to Eat to Have a Healthy Pregnancy by Trimester

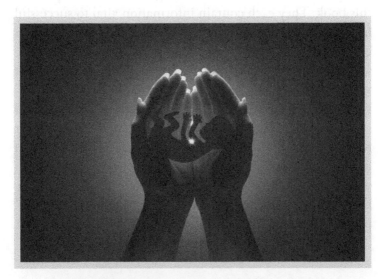

Source: Big Stock Photo.com. Used with permission.

> *"If I had my life to live over, instead of wishing away nine months of pregnancy, I'd have cherished every moment and realized that the wonderment growing inside me was the only chance in life to assist God in a miracle."*
>
> —*Erma Bombeck*

I went through two pregnancies, nineteen months apart, to bring my beautiful daughters into this world. I had early signals that each of my daughters would be her own person. They would share the same blood and the same heritage; they even looked a lot alike until they were a few years old. But wow, they had completely different personalities! I have always wondered if the distinct experiences I had during each pregnancy were a sign of their uniqueness.

During my first pregnancy, I had severe nausea all day long every day but had little trouble eating. In fact, eating seemed to resolve the nausea, unfortunately. During my second pregnancy, the nausea was much more manageable, but I had no appetite and lost ten pounds during the first trimester. Not to worry. I put the weight back on in spades through the remainder of my pregnancy. And there were other, adorable little signs of how different they would be. One rolled and tumbled throughout the months in vitro, the other kicked and punched. One was a relatively easy, completely natural birthing process. (It was very "in" at that time to not use any anesthesia or medications during delivery.) The other fought the process to the point where I thought she was trying to crawl back up inside me.

As a nutritionist, I now understand what I didn't know then—that my diet and probable nutrient deficiencies were at least partially responsible for some of the fairly dramatic changes in how I felt from one pregnancy to the next.

The one thing that was constant through both of my pregnancies was my tireless determination to devour as much information as I could find that would describe what was going on each new day and week of my journey. I loved looking at the images of how my growing baby looked at various stages. I counted the days when it would go from being an adorable little lima bean (embryo) to a fully developed fetus. I was fascinated at each step of organ development, and relished every new thing I was feeling...yes, the good and the not-so-good!

I wanted this chapter to give you a few images and graphical depictions similar to those that I found so captivating and engaging during my pregnancies. Along with the pictures, you will find a summary of fetal development for each trimester, physical and emotional changes occurring in mom, and specific nutritional considerations at each stage.

Pregnancy Changes Everything

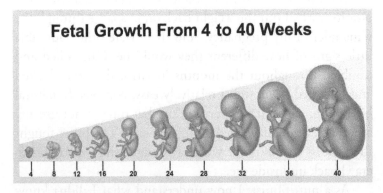

Fetal Growth From 4 to 40 Weeks

Source: BigStockPhoto.com. Used with permission.

Pregnancy changes a woman in almost every way. The baby bump, or belly, is by far the most fascinating aspect to the woman, and frankly, to those around her. The other changes going on, physical and emotional, are less perceptible, but equally profound.

There are digestive changes, changes to the urinary tract, breasts become sensitive and enlarged, the vulva becomes engorged, some women will notice an acceleration of hair and nail growth. There are many, many changes, including emotional ones, that are all considered healthy and normal.

Each woman's pregnancy will be different as will the degree to which some of these changes will be inconvenient, like having to pee more frequently or deal with extremely sensitive breasts. No matter what, most women agree that it is one of the most exciting life experiences they will ever have, and no wonder, considering the miracle that is beginning inside them.

Eating Healthy—First Trimester

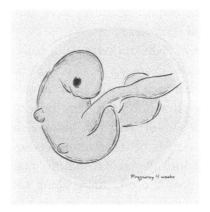

Source: BigStockPhoto.com. Used with permission.

A pregnancy kicks into gear when the sperm and ovum come together in the fallopian tube and fertilization takes place. As the egg grows, the zygote (fertilized egg) divides into a cluster of cells and finds its way to the uterus where, by the sixth day, it attaches itself to the uterine lining.[1] By the tenth or eleventh day following conception, the woman is indeed pregnant! By the end of the first two weeks, the placenta, which has the job of transferring nutrients from the mother to the baby as well as removing wastes from the baby, also develops.[2]

Fetal Development

From weeks three to seven, the developing baby is usually referred to as an embryo. A great deal of development occurs during this first several weeks, including all the baby's facial features, with large dark circles where the eyes will later develop. The mouth, lower jaw and throat are developing, blood cells form, and circulation begins. The tiny "heart," which is only a tube at this point, will beat about 65 times a minute by the end of the fourth week and can usually be detected around six weeks.[3]

During weeks eight to twelve, your baby's facial features will develop more. There is a small fold of skin on each side of the head where each ear will grow, as well as tiny "buds" that eventually grow into arms, legs, fingers, and toes. The neural tube consists of what will become the brain, spinal cord, and other parts of the central nervous system and is well developed into the second month. The digestive tract and sensory organs also take form, along with the development of bone to replace existing cartilage.[4] During this time your baby can open and close its fists and mouth. Fingernails and toenails are beginning to form, the circulatory and urinary systems are now working, and the liver is producing bile.[5] It is also possible to identify the gender of the baby around ten to twelve weeks. At the end of the first trimester, and your baby's most critical developmental period, it is now four inches and weighs about one ounce. Chances of miscarriage drop considerably after three months.[6]

Mom's Physical and Emotional Changes

By the fifteenth day following conception, when you might normally expect your period to begin, you may notice instead that your breasts are tender and have a feeling of fullness or bloating in your belly.[7] These sensations might even be normal for you just prior to your period starting. If you have been trying to get pregnant, you are carefully monitoring the days and hours to see if you are "late." Hormonal changes are affecting almost every organ in your body and can trigger symptoms even in the very early weeks of pregnancy.[8] Of course there are always a few women who won't even realize they are pregnant until their tummy is protruding so far it forces them to get checked out by a doctor. But according to WomensHealth.gov, most women will notice at least a couple of the following symptoms during the first trimester:

- Extreme tiredness
- Swollen breasts and nipples
- Upset stomach with or without vomiting
- Food cravings or loss of appetite
- Mood swings
- Constipation
- Frequent urination

- Headache
- Heartburn
- Weight gain or loss

(www.womenshealth.gov/pregnancy/
youre-pregnant-now-what/stages-pregnancy)

Mood changes are also common during the first trimester for many women. Some women will keep a lot of this to themselves because they think it's all in their imagination, but in fact, there are biochemical reasons that you're bursting into tears watching those puppy-rescue commercials on TV.

The significant changes that are occurring with a woman's hormones also affect the neurotransmitters in the brain, which are responsible for mood regulation. These changes can be further exacerbated by some of the other symptoms plaguing you, like excessive fatigue. The mood swings, like so many of the other symptoms that can pop up, are usually temporary. If your mood changes continue for more than two or three weeks, or they morph into full-blown anxiety or depression, check in with your healthcare practitioner and discuss what alternatives are available to you. Do not try to be the brave, stoic new mom. You have a beautiful little miracle, a new human life growing inside you. This is important enough to ask for help and advice if you need it. Some things require a team approach; this is one of them.

Many of these issues cause women to worry and wonder whether all of this is normal. It is. The good news is most of these early symptoms dissipate as your pregnancy progresses.

Try to view these things as temporary inconveniences; each one is a beautiful sign that your body is making the accommodations it needs to welcome your baby into your womb. Make necessary changes to your life whenever possible to accommodate how you're feeling. For instance, allow extra time in your schedule to rest if you're dealing with excessive tiredness, or make sure you have quick access to a restroom if you notice the need to urinate frequently.

Nutrition and Lifestyle Considerations

If you are following the plan in this book, you have already cleaned up your diet and your lifestyle so you can welcome your growing baby into the healthiest internal environment possible. A lot of toxins have already been removed. If you haven't taken these steps, now is definitely the time. As soon as you become suspicious that you may be pregnant, things like smoking and drinking alcohol should stop immediately. You should also avoid prescription drugs and over-the-counter medications that are not approved by your doctor.

Specific nutritional considerations during the first trimester include:

- Drink plenty of water—a minimum of ten cups (eighty ounces) per day. Optimal hydration while pregnant is critical because of the amount of fluid that will be absorbed by your developing baby. Without proper hydration, your body cannot detoxify and remove wastes effectively, cannot absorb nutrients, and cannot keep up with the production of plasma that is required by the placenta. Get yourself organized to track your daily water intake to help you stay on track.
- Eat foods rich in vitamin B6 or supplement with vitamin B6—women who experience nausea and/or

vomiting during the first trimester are often found to be deficient in vitamin B6.[9] Consume organic foods high in B6 including avocados, sunflower seeds, pistachios, walnuts, cashews, tuna, wild salmon, chicken, turkey, prunes, raisins, apricots, and lean grass-fed beef. If your nausea or vomiting is severe or prolonged, you should use a supplement form of B6 rather than wait until your natural reserves increase from food intake, which isn't going to happen overnight. Take a high-quality supplement made from real food sources that does not contain fillers or toxins. (Refer to Chapter 7 on Supplements.) Take only the recommended dosage.

- Eat high-fiber, high-protein foods. Fiber is beneficial to healthy bowel movements by correcting the bacteria in the gut and improving waste elimination. Protein will help stabilize blood sugar and help with food cravings. Focus your food choices on organic sources including poultry, lean grass-fed beef, eggs, wild-caught salmon or tuna, all types of beans, artichokes, peas, broccoli, brussels sprouts, legumes, raspberries, blackberries, avocados, pears. Add chia seeds and flaxseed meal to oatmeal, yogurt or smoothies.

- Drink ginger root tea or beet kvass. These are tea-like beverages that have liver-supporting properties to help with detoxification and elimination. They are also helpful in preventing nausea and vomiting during the first trimester. Also, other than supporting your body's natural detoxification process, any hardcore detoxification methods should be postponed until after you deliver and are done breastfeeding.

Constipation. Be sure you're drinking the proper amount of purified or filtered water if dealing with constipation. You can also try eating several smaller meals each day instead of the normal breakfast, lunch and dinner. Laxatives and most herbal supplements that would normally be used for constipation (such as aloe vera juice), are not recommended during pregnancy due to the risk of stimulating uterine constractions. If you are having a severe problem with constipation, speak to your healthcare provider for specific recommendations.

Eating Healthier—Second Trimester

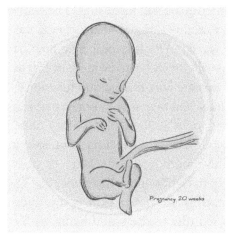

Source: BigStockPhoto.com. Used with permission

Fetal Development

Around the beginning of your second trimester (fourth month), your baby is now able to make sucking motions and facial expressions. The eyes are almost fully developed and the lids are fused closed while the rest of this development continues. Soft, downy hair will grow and begin to cover your baby's body. Your baby has fingerprints, nipples, and the back begins to straighten. The bones are hardening, and by your sixteenth week, your baby measures seven to eight inches in length and weighs around four ounces.[10] By five months the legs have reached their full length. When the baby moves and kicks, you will start to notice subtle yet often unmistakable sensations. In some cases the kicks and pokes won't be so subtle! You may also start to notice when your baby has the hiccups, which will feel like a series of "knocks" in your belly. Your little one can now suck his or her thumb, grab onto the umbilical cord, or even scratch his or her face. There is more hair on the head, and the eyebrows are formed although the eyes themselves are still fused shut. The baby's body is now covered with a creamy substance that protects the skin from the surrounding water.[11] The heartbeat may now be audible by a fetoscope and will usually be in the range of 120 to 160 beats per minute. The ears are fully formed and functional, and can hear plenty of sounds. You may start to notice that certain sounds—singing, yelling, quiet or loud music—may cause gentle movements from your baby; it is reacting to outside stimuli! By the end of the fifth month, your baby is ten or twelve inches long and weighs about eight ounces. Incredible!

At six months the baby's skin is translucent, wrinkled, and appears red due to the blood being visible through the skin.[12] Permanent tooth buds have formed, and hair growth is apparent. The eyes are developed and open around this time, and the baby can make both crying and sucking motions. The arm and leg muscles have developed and are getting stronger. If you try to tickle or grab your baby's foot it might just surprise you and pull away or kick you! At six months your baby is about twelve to fourteen inches long and weighs somewhere around one and a half pounds.[13]

Mom's Physical and Emotional Changes

Most women find the second trimester easier than the first, but it becomes even more important to pay attention to the care you are giving your body and that of your growing baby. By the beginning of the second trimester, your abdomen is starting to expand. Your uterus is about the size of a large grapefruit, and you should start to feel better from any nausea or general uncomfortable sensations or symptoms that have been occurring. But as those things subside, other changes slowly appear. According to U.S. Department of Health and WomensHealth.org, you may notice one or more of the following during your second trimester:

- Body aches, such as back, abdomen, groin, or thigh pain
- Stretchmarks may appear on your abdomen, breasts, thighs, or butt
- Darkening of the skin around your nipples
- A line will form on the skin between your belly button to the pubic hairline
- Patches of darker skin, usually over the cheeks, forehead, nose, or upper lip. Oftencalled the "mask of pregnancy."
- Numb or tingling hands (carpal tunnel syndrome)
- Itching on the abdomen, palms, and soles of feet. (If itching sensations are combined with nausea, loss of appetite, vomiting, jaundice, or fatigue, you should schedule a visit with your doctor. The combination of these symptoms can be a telltale sign of a liver issue that should be evaluated right away.)

(www.womenshealth.gov/pregnancy/
youre-pregnant-now-what/stages-pregnancy)

Nutrition Considerations

- Eat foods high in healthy fats.
- Stick with organic whenever possible; minimize intake of toxins.
- Increase intake of organic fruits and vegetables.
- Continue drinking plenty of water. Adequate hydration is critical throughout your pregnancy—preferably purified, distilled, or filtered water. Do not count fruit juices, sugary drinks, or flavored water toward your fluid tracking.

Still Eating Healthy—Third Trimester

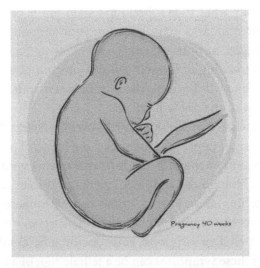

BigStockPhoto.com. Used with permission.

The anticipation and excitement has been building for many months now—you are in the homestretch! This is a good time to finish any preparations for the nursery, finalize your list of names, and take a new baby class. Most importantly, this is a time to focus on you. Spend time with your significant other and loved ones, get plenty of rest and relaxation, spend time talking to your baby and playing relaxing music for him or her, and of course continue your focus on staying well nourished.

Fetal Development

During the final trimester, your baby will start to gain weight rapidly and store vital minerals such as iron and calcium.[14] At seven months the lungs, although not fully formed, can function at a minimal level outside the uterus, and may occasionally perform practice "breathing." It is at this point that your baby could survive if born prematurely.[15] The baby now sees the sunlight through your abdomen and may react to bright light by attempting to turn away from it. Around eight months the baby's skin is losing the wrinkles it had earlier in the pregnancy. The baby has less and less space to move around so his or her movements seem less forceful. Instead of kicking, you will notice more stretching, turning, and wiggling. The hair that once covered the baby's entire body is starting to lessen and will continue to do so until birth. The baby is between sixteen and eighteen inches in length, and weight will range between four and seven pounds.

At nine months, your baby has reached full maturity. Your job as a nurturing host for the creation of this new life is coming to its natural, miraculous conclusion very soon. Your baby is nearly ready for life in the outside world!

All the senses are well formed; the organs are ready to function independently of your body. The wrinkles have all disappeared, and the baby's head will begin to settle into your pelvis. Your baby is now around nineteen to twenty-one inches long and is close to its final birth weight, around six to nine pounds.

Mom's Physical and Emotional Changes

Some women become physically uncomfortable into the third trimester. As described above, your baby is getting large and starts to crowd the abdominal cavity, not leaving a lot of room for your organs. When I was pregnant, I waited anxiously for the day when I could no longer see my toes without bending forward. For me that was a milestone that signified that I was almost to the finish line. Whatever your "milestone" is, pay attention because it's approaching fast now!

Mood changes often resurface during the third trimester, as can nausea or sometimes even vomiting. In addition to the challenges of simply moving around, you may start to notice things like difficulty breathing, issues with heartburn, trouble sleeping, hemorrhoids, or swelling of the ankles, fingers, and toes. (Sudden or extreme swelling or weight gain should be reported immediately to your doctor, and may indicate preeclampsia.)[16] It's fairly common for most women to report a very frequent need to urinate during the final month or two of pregnancy. The baby's size is putting lots of pressure on your bladder, so the frequent trips to the bathroom are to be expected. Your baby is also generating lots of heat which may cause you to feel an increase in your own skin temperature. Below are a few other changes highlighted on the Johns Hopkins Medicine website:[17]

- Your blood pressure may decrease as the fetus presses on the main vein that returns blood to the heart.

- Hair may start to grow on your arms, legs, and face due to increased hormone stimulation of hair follicles. Your hair may also become courser in texture.
- You may experience leg cramps.
- Stretch marks may appear or darken.
- Colostrum may begin to leak from your nipples in preparation for breastfeeding.
- Your sex drive may decrease.
- Backaches may occur or intensify.
- Hemorrhoids may develop or become more severe.
- Varicose veins in the legs may develop or become more painful.

The other changes occurring in the woman's body toward the end of the third trimester are signs that it is preparing to give birth. If you are using a traditional doctor, obstetrician, or midwife, they usually will start internal vaginal exams to determine if your cervix is thinning or softening (called "effacing"). This is a normal process that helps the birth canal to open for the birthing process.

Nutrition Considerations

- Eat small frequent meals instead of three large meals each day. Due to the size of your baby in the eighth and ninth months, it is likely putting pressure on your stomach, making it difficult to eat and digest large quantities of food in one sitting.
- Eat high-quality protein from organic sources—organic nuts, eggs, meat, poultry, and fish. Protein requirements for mother's during the third trimester double to eighty to one hundred grams a day so your

body can support your needs as well as the needs of your baby. Remember: It is during the third trimester that your baby is rapidly gaining much-needed fat tissues and weight. Proteins are the building blocks of all tissues in the body. You will want to be well fortified so there's plenty from which your baby can draw.

- Eat foods high in fiber from organic sources. Fruits and vegetables help move digested particles through the digestive tract, help with constipation, and provide much-needed nutrients to support all biological and metabolic processes for you and your baby.
- Maintain fluid intake at a minimum of ten cups (eighty ounces) per day. The best fluids by far are purified or filtered water. Acceptable fluids do not include sugary drinks, flavored water, or fruit juices—all are loaded with sugar, which you definitely don't need or want at this stage.

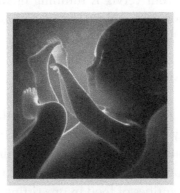

Source: Shutterstock.com. Used with permission.

ABSOLUTELY
NO
ALCOHOL
BEYOND
THIS POINT

Don't Mess with Your Hormones: Important Things to Avoid during Pre-conception and Pregnancy

"I come from a family where gravy is considered a beverage."

—*Erma Bombeck*

Foods and lifestyle factors that would typically be considered by most of us to be "healthy" or normal often increase the risk factors for infertility, poor fetal development, and compromised health of your newborn when consumed regularly or in excess. Some of these are mentioned in other areas of the book, but are repeated again in this section to make it easy for you to reference.

As you start reading through this list, you may hear your inner voice screaming in horror saying, "No way, I'm not gonna give up *that*!" But if you truly want to have a healthy pregnancy, or, more importantly, if you have been unable to conceive, you will want to take each one of these recommendations seriously and get these things out of your mouth and your life.

Similar to the Pre-Conception Strategy for Men and Women, you will want to use a time frame of six to eight months to have each of these items 100 percent eliminated. That is, you want six to eight months free and clear of the things listed below to give your body time to repair, heal, and, hopefully, get your fertility hormones charged up and raring to go.

Foods to Avoid

Artificial sweeteners. Avoid all artificial sweeteners including diet sweeteners and foods labeled sugar-free. These are manufactured with toxic chemicals that disrupt hormone signaling, cause inflammation, and disrupt digestion.[1]

Fish. Avoid fish that contain mercury—specifically swordfish, shark, mackerel, and tilefish—during pregnancy, or more generally for women during childbearing age. These fish are often found to contain high levels of methyl-mercury, a powerful human neurotoxin that easily crosses the placenta and has the potential to damage the fetal nervous system.[2] Babies who are exposed to mercury during pregnancy can suffer brain damage as well as hearing and vision problems.[3] It's best to limit other seafood consumption, including tuna, to no more than once per week during pre-conception and pregnancy.

Bitter melon. Bitter melon is a green cucumber-shaped fruit (sometimes used as a vegetable) that is usually available in the fall. Some would say it is an ugly version of a cucumber. It is low in calories, an excellent source of several nutrients, and has been used for centuries as treatment for various health conditions. But bitter melon also contains substances that have been shown to stimulate uterine contractions, possibly causing pre-term labor.[4]

Caffeine. Coffee, soda, and tea. Caffeine depletes the body of nutrients and hydration, both of which can become dangerous during pregnancy if caffeine is consumed in large quantities on a regular basis.[5]

Processed and refined foods, fast food, and "junk food." Eliminate as many foods as possible that contain toxic chemicals, fillers, sugars, preservatives, and artificial ingredients. When eating out, seek out restaurants that are advertising and implementing a health food strategy, or better yet, an organic food strategy. See the list below for specific foods to avoid that would be considered "processed."

Trans fats, partially hydrogenated fats. Commonly used by fast-food restaurants to prepare food and found in pre-packaged foods, fried foods in restaurants, cake mixes, pancake mixes, and ice cream. Most of these substances will be eliminated when you stop eating processed and refined foods. Read food labels. These fats are known to accumulate in the body and reduce the healthy fat content of breast milk, as well as increase your bad cholesterol levels and contribute to type 2 diabetes.[6]

Non-organic dairy products. Dairy products are known to cause inflammation and play havoc with your hormones. On average, dairy products account for 60–70 percent of estrogens consumed.[7] In fact, numerous other hormones have been found in cow's milk, including prolactin, melatonin, oxytocin, insulin, and progesterone.[8] These hormones, along with other chemicals (up to twenty) from the homogenizing process, are known to contribute to inflammation in the body and be risk factors for ear, nose, and throat infections in children whose parents consumed them on a regular basis.[9] Consuming dairy products that are made from cows fed with hormone additives can disrupt the endocrine system, leading to hormonal imbalances, which can cause male infertility as well as Polycystic Ovary Syndrome and endometriosis in women.[10]

Herbs and Spices to Avoid

Saffron. Avoid foods that contain saffron. Saffron is a spice found in the purple crocus flower. Modern research shows it is useful as an antioxidant, anti-inflammatory, and has anticancer properties. Despite these benefits, it is generally not recommended for use during pregnancy or nursing due to safety concerns if used in large doses. In amounts as small as two tablespoons, it can be narcotic, toxic and even lethal, causing violent hemorrhages.[11]

Sage. Avoid foods that contain sage during pregnancy and nursing. Although it is regarded as a powerful antioxidant, it is also known prevent perspiration and dries up the flow of milk during lactation.[12]

Excessive salt. Salt is an important nutrient during pregnancy, but will cause an imbalance with other vitamin and mineral levels if excess amounts are consumed on a regular basis.[13]

Other herbs. There are many other herbs and spices that should be used with caution or only under the supervision of a qualified herbalist. Below are some of the more common from this list that should be avoided during pregnancy.[14]

Aloe, aloe vera	Juniper Berries
Arnica	Licorice
Barberry	Lily of the Valley
Blue cohosh	Mistletoe
Butternut	Nutmeg
Calendula	Parsley (small amounts are okay)
Comfrey	Periwinkle
Feverfew	Rhubarb
Ginseng	Wormwood
Goldenseal	

Lifestyle Issues to Avoid

Dehydration. Purified or filtered water should continue to be your primary source of hydration. Proper hydration is necessary to avoid neural tube defects, low amniotic fluid, inadequate breast milk production, premature labor, and poor development of the placenta.

Nicotine. Most traditional OB/GYN physicians will strongly caution a pregnant woman about the health hazards smoking causes for her and her baby. It is known to cause asthma and recurrent ear, nose and throat infections in children who were born from one or both parents who smoked. What is not usually mentioned or known to couples who are thinking of becoming pregnant is that both the man and the woman should stop smoking at least three months before conception.[15] Smoking in the three months before conception can damage the DNA in sperm, impact the development of the ovaries, cause premature aging of a woman's eggs, cause childhood leukemia, and also reduces fertility in moms and dads.[16] Research has shown that stopping a minimum of three months prior to conception gives your cells and tissues enough time to recuperate from the damage and create a healthier internal environment for conception and fetal development.[17]

No dieting. Much to the horror of many women, weight gain during pregnancy is normal and necessary to accommodate the growing life inside you. Once pregnant, the time for eating healthy has begun, but the time for "dieting" (a reduced-calorie diet) is over. Reducing your caloric intake has major health consequences for the mother and the developing baby if conception has already occurred. Any weight issues that exist prior to conception should be dealt with several months before trying to conceive. Restricting the intake of nutritious foods after conception has occurred will cause the fetus to use protein and other nutrients from the mother's body, potentially causing difficulties during labor and delivery.[18]

Never Detoxify or Cleanse during Pregnancy. Implementing steps to increase the natural detoxification process in the body can be very beneficial in improving health, but only in an individual who is not pregnant or currently breastfeeding. Taking special supplements or large quantities of detoxifying foods increases the cleansing process in the body, which consumes energy and vital nutrients that would otherwise be directed to supporting pregnancy or nourishing a mother's milk. Many new moms are desperate to have their body return to normal and lose the pregnancy weight. Don't do it. Your body needs to heal, cells need to be replaced, and tissues need to regenerate. Ultimately, you will do more harm than good to your health by trying to fast-track your way back into your skinny jeans.

Drugs. Recreational drugs, pharmaceutical medicines, aspirin or cannabis (Marijuana) all contribute to infertility, stunted fetus growth, below-average IQ in children exposed during pregnancy, and other complications. Marijuana contains a fertility toxin, cannabinoid, which has been shown to cause problems in men and women. In women, it can impair cell-signaling pathways, alter hormone regulation, and cause problems with embryo implantation. In men, cannabinoids have been found to inhibit testosterone production, reduce energy production in sperm, decrease sperm motility ("swimming" capabilities), and decrease sperm function.[19] In addition to these inherent problems with marijuana, it is often contaminated with herbicides and pesticides, which are toxic to the human body and quickly absorbed into the body when inhaled.[20] Talk to your physician before discontinuing any medications that were prescribed specifically for you.

Unnecessary medications. If you are taking any prescription medications, work with your doctor to determine if it is necessary for you to continue it while pregnant. Avoid over-the-counter medications as well. Medications, such as Tylenol, Advil, Excedrin, cold and flu remedies, antacids, laxatives, and anti-diarrhea medications, when used frequently, all have their drawbacks and potential risks during pregnancy. Check with your obstetrician before taking anything other than your supplements and prenatal vitamin.

Stress. Stress puts a greater demand on the body for nutrients; we burn up more when we are in a stress response. This is particularly important during pre-conception. Stress activates a response from the adrenal glands, which also impacts hormone regulation and can interfere with fertility and conception.[21]

Alcohol. Alcohol should be avoided during pre-conception and pregnancy. As little as one drink can lead to a 50 percent reduction in conception.[22] Frequent or excessive alcohol consumption is associated with hormone imbalance, irregular menstrual cycle, and is strongly linked to miscarriage. When consumed during pregnancy or in excess prior to conception, it is known to create a greater risk for retardation, hyperactivity, deformities, and heart problems in a newborn child, as well as difficulties in later developmental stages.[23]

Xenoestrogens. Xenoestrogens are substances that mimic the effects of natural estrogen and disrupt the body's natural hormone balance. Research has shown that xenoestrogens are often contributing factors in miscarriages, infertility, and birth defects.[24] They are typically found in items such as plastic containers used for storing, heating, and microwaving foods (Soft, pliable plastics are the worst offenders.). Be sure not to heat *anything* in plastic. They can also be found in, non-organic cleaning supplies, packaged foods that contain dyes and preservatives, cosmetics, and hair products, garden pesticides and non-organic meats and dairy products.[25]

Correct Issues with Oral Hygiene. Signs of poor oral hygiene should be resolved two to three months prior to conception. Women with poor oral health, specifically gum disease, can take, on average, two months longer to get pregnant than women without gum disease.[26] Other studies have shown that a woman with gum disease is more likely to have a pre-term birth and impaired fetal growth.[27] Regular brushing and flossing, along with intake of vitamin C and a good anti-oxidant such as CoQ10, are effective in supporting good oral hygiene.

Don't Drink Unfiltered Tap Water. Our public water systems are being constantly polluted by industrial waste, byprod-ucts, pharmaceutical drugs, pesticides, herbicides, and com-mercial cleaning products.[28] Even if you have a private well as your water source, it should be checked for heavy metal contamination before drinking its water.

To make sure you are clear about your food choices, below is a detailed list of many processed, high-sugar, gluten-con-taining, inflammatory foods that I strongly urge you to elim-inate or dramatically reduce (no more than three servings per week) in your weekly diet. This is particularly important for anyone trying to resolve an existing inflammatory condition (like gum disease or irritable bowel syndrome), infections such as sinus or chronic UTIs, or other health condition such as obesity, blood sugar imbalance, or chronic stress.

Processed (Man-Made) Carbohydrates
Your goal is to eliminate all man-made (processed) carbohydrates.

Remember: You should eat real, fresh, organic carbohydrates whenever possible. Please read labels and remember to avoid all processed or packaged carbohydrates that have partially hydrogenated and/or hydrogenated fats. (See "Avoid" list above.)

Breads

Bread crumbs (unless gluten-free)	Oat bran bread	Wheatberry
	Oatmeal bread	Whole-grain
Corn tortilla	Pumpernickel	Raisin bread
Cracked-wheat bread	bread	Whole-grain pita
	Rice bran bread	Whole-grain or
Cracker meal	Rye bread	7-grain bread
Breads (unless gluten-free)	Wheat bran bread	
	Wheat germ bread	

Crackers

Crackers are considered a processed food that you will want to eliminate completely or consume in very small amounts, and only if gluten-free. Even the so-called "healthy" products (such as those listed below) will contain many additives, including hydrogenated fats.

Rice cakes	Rusk toast	Wheat Euphrates
Rye wafers (wasa)	Rye crispbread	Wheat melba toast
Rice crackers	Wheat crackers (Ak-mak)	Whole-wheat matzo

Processed Snack Foods

Beef jerky
Corn chips
Corn nuts
Meat-based sticks

Pizza
Pork skins
Popcorn
Potato chips

Pretzels
Sesame sticks
Taro chips
Trail mix

Processed Foods

Canned foods
Dried soups

Fast Foods
Mixes

Packaged foods

Condiments
(Contain Sugar and Chemical Additives)

Barbecue sauces
Fish sauces
Gravies
Hoisin sauce

Ketchup
Meat extender
Meat tenderizer
Oyster sauce

Relishes
Sweet pickles
Worcestershire sauce

Sugar and Desserts
(Contain Sugar and Chemical Additives)

Banana chips
Fruit butters
Processed yogurt
(low-fat, non-
fat or flavored)
Brown sugar
Fruit leathers
Pudding
Cakes

Gelatin desserts
Sherbet
Candy
Granola
Snack or
breakfast bars
Frosting
Protein bars

Caramel flavored
popcorn
Honey
Ice cream
Strudel
Cheesecake
Jams, jellies,
preserves,
marmalade

High-fructose corn, caramel, sorghum, syrups
Cocoa
Milkshakes

Toaster pastries
Cookies
Molasses
White sugar
Doughnuts

Pastries
Eclairs
Pie
Sweet rolls
Frozen desserts

Man-Made or Refined Grain Products

Bagels
Flour tortillas
Pizza dough
Banana bread
French bread
Popovers
Biscuits
Ice cream cone
Puff pastry
Bread sticks
Irish soda bread

Scones
Chinese noodles
Macaroni
Waffles
Cold cereal
Muffins
White English muffins
Corn cakes
Navajo bread
White rice

Cornbread stuffing
Noodles
White hamburger buns
Cream of rice
Pancakes
Wonton wrappers
Dinner rolls
Phyllo dough

High Processed/Cured Meat and Sausages

Don't eat cured meats, including bacon, hot dogs, jerky, or ham. They contain sodium nitrate and/or sodium nitrites which are compounds that keep food from spoiling and dramatically increase your risk of cancer by combining with amino acids from other foods in the stomach to form highly carcinogenic compounds.

Bacon
Ham
Pastrami

Barbecue loaf
Hot dogs
Peppered loaf

Beer salami
Honey loaf
Pepperoni

Beerwurst   Bologna   Corned beef loaf
Honey-roll sausage   Lebanon bologna   Mother's loaf
Picnic loaf   Port headcheese   Salami
Vienna sausage

Fats That Contain Damaged Fats, Chemicals and/or Sugar

Bottled salad   Shortening   Whipped cream
dressing   Cream substitutes   (and other
Margarine   Palm oil   dessert toppings)
Sandwich spreads   Sour cream   High-fat meats
Buttermilk   (imitation)   (cooked at
Mayonnaise   Deep-fat   high temperatures)
(imitation)   fried foods   Half-and-half

CHAPTER 8

Healthy Mom, Happy Baby: Recommendations for Post-Pregnancy Diet and Health

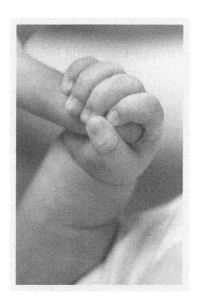

Source: BigStockPhoto.com. Used with permission.

*"Perhaps this is the moment for
which you were created."*

—*Esther 4:14*

Bringing Home Baby—A Reality Check

I'm going to tell you a secret. It's not the type of secret I need you to keep to yourself (obviously), but the type that is meant to offer you comfort on the day you become a new mom. Most moms, or dads for that matter, will rarely admit that they dealt with what I'm about to tell you, but I think it's fairly common.

Here it is: I was terrified to bring my firstborn home from the hospital. I mean, terrified with a capital T.

Don't misunderstand; I was beyond thrilled to finally have her in my life after months of anticipation…nine months of a normal but fascinating pregnancy. But in spite of the optimism I felt over my future life as a mom, now I was bringing my little bundle of joy home with me for the first time. Everything from dressing her in the hospital, to getting her into the car, not yet adept at juggling baby paraphernalia and a baby—it all seemed so awkward that I felt embarrassed and conspicuous. I felt as if everyone *knew* I didn't know what I was doing! The embarrassment turned to panic—it welled up inside me like a geyser ready to burst as I entered our apartment with her in my arms. We dropped on the dining room table all the stuff the hospital sends home with you, looked down at the little angel sleeping in my arms and thought, *What the hell do we do now?*

I had a wonderful, healthy, "normal" experience with labor and delivery. I was very lucky that was the case because

I had gained 50 pounds by the time I delivered. (Remember: As I confessed in Chapter 2, my dietary staple during pregnancy was hot fudge brownie sundaes.)

My labor was 100 percent drug-free, which was the popular thing to do at that time, so it was intense in terms of dealing with contractions without anesthesia. My delivery was also very normal; about 45 minutes of pushing and I had my beautiful, six-pound six-ounce little girl in my arms. Oh my god, she was a beauty! I'll never forget how calm she seemed given what she had just endured. No crying. She just laid there in my arms, staring directly into my eyes as if to say, "There you are!"

I couldn't have been more overjoyed as a new, first-time mom. But secretly, deep inside, I harbored fears about not really knowing how to take care of this precious little soul. At the same time, I didn't understand how I would ever get back to the life I use to know.

As we stood there in our apartment, my husband and I realized that we were both sort of frozen. "This is silly," we both agreed. "Let's just go about our normal routine." Yeah, right. "Normal" was gone. Meanwhile, as the minutes after our arrival ticked on, I was getting more anxious about a whole litany of things, each one seeming more monumental than the last.

Should I lay her down in her crib and wait until she lets me know what she needs? How will she let me know? Should I just sit in a chair until she cries? Is it okay for me to go wash the dishes in the sink? What do I do when I need to use the bathroom and can't get to her quickly if she starts crying? What about all those little baby noises I'm hearing, are those normal? And each time I hear a baby noise my breasts fill up with milk and start leaking through *everything*, what's that about?

Sure, I read books. I studied the Lamaze method of natural childbirth and breastfeeding. I even took a few classes on caring for a newborn that our hospital offered to expecting parents. I thought I was ready,but somehow reading about all of this and *experiencing* it are two very different things. No one warned me about the panic, insecurity, and worry that sets in; the realization that this newly minted life is 100 percent dependent on me and my ability to make sound decisions for her care.

I've had plenty of years to reflect on those memories. I made my mistakes; everyone does. You will too, but overall, they are wonderful, cherished memories. No matter what amount of worry or panic takes you over in the beginning, know that it is more normal than people will admit. After all, those little cuties don't exactly come out waving an instruction manual in your face!

I'm convinced that being a little bit insecure or unsure of your future as a new parent is all part of becoming a new parent. Parenting is full of the unexpected.

You can't possibly be prepared for every nuance. No matter how many books you read or what lengths you go to acquire every speck of knowledge about newborns or child-rearing, your baby will most certainly come up with a little noise, behavior, food sensitivity, rash, or schedule anomaly that will be a mystery to moms everywhere.

Everything you experience with your child is new for them and new for you. You will face each new thing—even the big ones—with confidence. You will trust your instincts. There is a "knowing" that comes from deep within. The incredible love and devotion you have for your baby will help guide you. When you feel a little overwhelmed, you'll read books, do research on the internet, and spend countless hours on the phone with your parents, sisters, other family members, and friends. But when all the worry is done, you too will have a home full of beautiful memories.

Getting Back to Normal—Don't Rush It

Having things return to "normal" becomes important and desirable to many women after giving birth. You may find yourself craving your old routines and habits with things like your sleep schedule, meal schedules, energy and mood levels, and of course at the top of the list is losing the pregnancy weight.

Giving birth to a new human being is one of the most inspiring and miraculous events you will ever experience. It is also one of the most biologically unmerciful achievements in terms of its impact on your body.

For nine months a woman's muscles, skeletal frame, and internal organs bear the increasing weight and drain on internal resources from the growing baby inside her. During a vaginal birth, muscles and other tissues stretch and sometimes tear as the baby is not-so-gently forced through the birth canal and vaginal opening. It is not uncommon for a bone here or there to sustain fractures due to the stress on them.[1]

In August, 2015, a study was published in the American Journal of Obstetrics & Gynecology in which the researchers compared childbirth to running a marathon, except the trauma inflicted on a woman's body is sudden and not preceded by months of training during which the body has time to adapt.[2] Their research showed that 29 percent of women had evidence of fractures in their pubic bones, while 41 percent had undiagnosed tears in pelvic floor muscles.[3] Having a baby is hard work, and even though we wouldn't have it any other way, it takes a toll on a woman's body.

There is no shortcut to healing from childbirth. Your fastest route to the old you is to keep yourself as healthy as possible.

Below I have grouped general health and nutrition recommendations in a timeline that begins after childbirth.

Early Days after Delivery

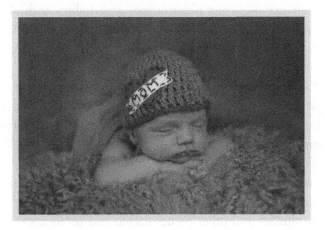

Source: BigStockPhoto.com. Used with permission.

During the initial days after giving birth, your body goes into full recovery mode. You may have lost a lot of blood and fluids during delivery. Your labor and delivery may have gone on over a period of many hours, so you will definitely be sleep-deprived and lacking energy. Your body will be sore and even swollen in places. This is a time to relax, rest, and enjoy whatever peaceful moments you have. Reflect on all you have been through over the last nine months and the beautiful future that awaits you. If you are lucky enough to receive offers of help—having meals delivered, help caring for your newborn or with chores around the house—accept as many as you can any and rest, rest, rest!

Now that your baby has arrived, it is very tempting to resume your old lifestyle and eating habits. Don't! Your body requires hydration and foods dense with nutrients as much now as ever. Continue drinking half your weight in ounces of purified, distilled, or filtered water every day. Eighty to ninety percent of all meals and snacks should be from organic, whole-food sources (not processed or fast food). Avoid alcohol consumption completely, and caffeine should stay at a maximum of two cups per day—especially important if you are breastfeeding. Maintain a diet of 60–70 percent non-starchy vegetables, 25 percent protein, and approximately 5 percent gluten-free grains.

Summary—Early Days after Delivery

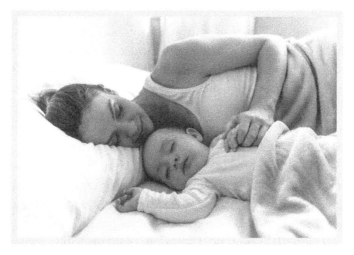

Source: BigStockPhoto.com. Used with permission.

- The three Rs: rest, relax, reflect.
- Carefully follow post-delivery instructions from your healthcare provider.
- Accept help with household chores.
- Drink half your body weight in ounces of purified, distilled, or filtered water every day. (e.g. if you weigh 140 pounds, you should drink about 70 ounces per day)
- Eighty to ninety percent of meals and snacks should come from organic, whole food sources.
- Avoid alcohol and caffeine; consume no more than two cups per day of caffeine, especially while breastfeeding.
- Keep food intake to 60–70 percent non-starchy vegetables, 25 percent protein, and 5 percent gluten-free grains.

Up to Six Weeks after Delivery

Your uterus will start to contract fairly soon after you deliver. These contractions can be very noticeable and sometimes painful. The rest of your internal organs, which all get shifted around during pregnancy, slowly return to their normal positions. Your pelvis is also recovering and returning to its pre-labor state as are your urethra, vagina, and anus. You may also have some bleeding at times following delivery.

You will most likely receive instructions from your obstetrician or midwife on how to keep stitches clean if you have them. If soreness persists, salt baths with lavender or calendula compresses can help reduce inflammation.

If you delivered by C-section, you probably received additional restrictions you will need to follow during the first few weeks after childbirth. Common things to avoid include climbing stairs, driving, or lifting anything heavier than your baby. Follow the advice of your doctor or midwife.

Whether you had a C-section or vaginal birth, it is usually advisable to keep activity levels to a minimum during these initial weeks after delivery. Any intense activity could impede the healing process. Limit activity to walking and gentle stretching to slowly recondition muscles.

Although rare, be aware of complications that can occur such as hemorrhoids, mastitis (Breast tissue becomes inflamed—red, sore, warm to the touch.), persistent back ache, or excessive sleep-deprivation. If any of these things occur or worsen, consult your healthcare provider.

You will likely feel fatigued during these weeks, especially if you are breastfeeding or your baby is not sleeping for extended periods of time. Incorporating deep-breathing sessions into your day can help minimize stress. Even three to five minutes, two or three times per day helps muscles to relax, delivers oxygen to the brain, helps lower blood pressure, releases endorphins, and stimulates detoxification processes.

Plenty of iron-rich foods such as dark leafy green vegetables, red meat, and poultry will help maintain adequate iron levels in your blood. Continue to avoid processed foods, foods high in sugar, and sugary beverages such as flavored waters, soda, or fruit juices. Continue drinking half your body weight in ounces of purified, distilled, or filtered water every day. Eighty to ninety percent of all meals and snacks should be from organic, whole food sources (i.e. nuts and seeds, organic fruits, avocado slices, gluten-free crackers). Avoid alcohol consumption and excessive caffeine (maximum two cups per day), especially important if you are breastfeeding. Maintain a diet of 60–70 percent non-starchy vegetables, 25 percent protein, and approximately 5 percent gluten-free grains.

Summary—Up to Six Weeks after Delivery

- Use salt water baths or calendula compresses for any residual inflammation or soreness.
- Continue to follow post-delivery instructions from your healthcare provider, especially following C-section.
- Deep breathing three to five minutes two to three times per day helps relieve stress, stimulates detoxification and healing, and lowers blood pressure.
- Drink half your body weight in ounces of purified, distilled, or filtered water every day.
- Eight to ninety percent of meals and snacks should come from organic, whole-food sources.
- Avoid alcohol and caffeine; consume no more than two cups per day of caffeine, especially while breastfeeding.
- Keep food intake to 60–70 percent non-starchy vegetables, 25 percent antibiotic-free and hormone-free protein, and 5 percent gluten-free grains.

Seven Weeks to Four Months after Delivery or Post-Breastfeeding

Most pregnancy hormones stay in your body until up to four months after you have discontinued breastfeeding. Any associated symptoms, such as pelvis or joint instability, can also continue for this amount of time. Continue limiting activities until you have been cleared by your doctor. Focus on yoga, Pilates, walking, or light resistance training.

During breastfeeding and for a while after, your body continues to store fat which is critical for hormone and milk production. Your hormones eventually get the message that breastfeeding has stopped, but give it time. Your body has innate healing abilities and is very wise.

Hopefully you are inspired to continue with the "clean," organic, whole-foods approach to nutrition to which, by now, you have grown accustomed, both in your daily eating habits and in your biochemistry. If you begin to treat yourself now and then to your favorite dessert, bread or pasta with dinner, a glass or two of wine, and the like, it is likely you will feel the effects by way of a headache, lethargy, digestive upset, or even a bout or two of diarrhea. Regularly adding "junk" foods back into your diet will also slow down the healing process that is occurring. A lot has happened over the weeks since delivering your baby. You are starting to feel back to the old you, and your household is acclimating nicely to your new family dynamic, but internally the healing is ongoing for several more months.

To continue supporting healthy eating and the healing process, stay focused on vegetables and dark leafy greens as the biggest food group you consume every day. High-quality, grass-fed meats and poultry, wild-caught seafood, gluten-free grains and organic fruits will help you maintain optimal health status. Continue to avoid processed foods, foods high in sugar, sugary beverages such as flavored waters, soda or fruit juices. Drinking half your body weight in ounces of purified, distilled, or filtered water every day is a habit you should continue for the rest of your life. Eighty to ninety percent of all meals and snacks should be from organic, whole food sources (i.e., nuts and seeds, organic fruits, avocado slices, gluten-free crackers). If you are done breastfeeding and would like to have an alcoholic beverage, stick with clear liquors, no soda or diet-soda mixers, avoid beer and flavored liquors. Maintain a diet of 60–70 percent non-starchy vegetables, 25 percent high-quality protein; and approximately 5 percent gluten-free grains and a small amount of low-glycemic fruit.

Summary—Seven Weeks to Four Months after Delivery

- Continue limiting activity until cleared by your doctor.
- Focus exercise to yoga, Pilates, walking, or light resistance training (again, if cleared by your doctor).
- Continue with healthy eating—focus on vegetables and dark leafy greens for the majority of food intake.
- Now okay to add an occasional treat—dessert, bread, or pasta on occasion, or even a glass or two of wine if you are done breastfeeding.
- Drink half your body weight in ounces (e.g. 140 pounds = 70 ounces) of purified, distilled, or filtered water every day.
- Eighty to ninety percent of meals and snacks should come from organic, whole food sources
- Maintain a diet of 60–70 percent non-starchy vegetables, 25 percent antibiotic-free and hormone-free protein, and approximately 5 percent gluten-free grains. Add in a small amount of low-glycemic fruit to your daily diet.

Four Months to One Year after Delivery

Even though most doctors will give you the all-clear, thumbs-up, you're-good-to-go sign way back at your six-week postpartum checkup, researchers advise otherwise. The University of Salford in the UK released findings in 2012 that it takes a year for a woman's body to completely heal from childbirth.[4] The idea that after a mere six weeks from delivery, a woman's body has recovered, is "pure fantasy" according to Doctor Wray.[5]

Do your own self-assessment and manage your nutrition and lifestyle in a manner that continues to support the subtle but ongoing healing that is yet to occur. If you notice residual achiness, pelvic pain, pain with intercourse, tiredness, mood swings, depression, constipation, or other symptoms, those are signs that your body is not fully recovered.

Being realistic here, with a new baby at home you do not have the luxury of treating yourself to frequent days of rest and leisure. Somewhere between four and twelve months from your delivery, many of you will have already jumped on the "Super-Mom" track and are barely coming up for air. Feeling tired? Of course you are! Who wouldn't feel tired with the physical and emotional demands you have taken on immediately after bringing a new human life into the world!

This is the time when your body is vulnerable to the onset of other health conditions, making it more important than ever to be taking care of yourself, paying attention to how you're feeling, and maintaining a nutritious, organic, whole-foods diet to support health, detoxification, and further healing. Any ongoing symptoms should be reported and evaluated by your healthcare practitioner.

Summary—Four Months to One Year after Delivery

- Even with the all-clear from your healthcare provider, it is likely your body is not done healing. Do your own self-assessment and manage your nutrition and lifestyle to support your continued recovery.

- Pay attention to signs of residual achiness, pelvic pain, pain with intercourse, tiredness, mood swings, depression, constipation, or other symptoms— these are signs that your body is not fully recovered. Significant depression or pain should be reported to your doctor.

- Be realistic with your time and schedule. If tiredness persists, schedule time for rest as often as you can.

- Drink half your body weight in ounces of purified, distilled, or filtered water every day (e.g. 140 pounds of weight = 70 ounces of water)

- Limit other beverages to two cups per day of caffeine, and as a general practice, stay away from sugary beverages such as fruit juices and soda.

- Eighty to ninety percent of meals and snacks should come from organic, whole food sources

- Maintain a diet of 60–70 percent non-starchy vegetables, 25 percent antibiotic-free and hormone-free protein, and approximately 5 percent gluten-free grains. Add in a small amount of low-glycemic fruit to your daily diet.

One to Two Years following Delivery

During pregnancy, your abdominal wall stretches. To assist with the stretching or lengthening process, your body responds by creating new muscle cells. Many experts believe it can take up to two years for the abdominal muscles to fully recover. There are three major factors that can slow down this recovery: (1) having a second pregnancy within two years of delivering your first; (2) gaining a large amount of weight during pregnancy; or (3) having a C-section (can cause scarring or adhesions in the abdominal tissues).

Summary—One to Two Years following Delivery

- Resume normal activities and exercise routine unless told otherwise by your doctor.
- Abdominal weakness can be addressed with regular stretching and exercise, but go easy if discomfort continues.
- Drink half your body weight in ounces in purified, distilled, or filtered water every day. (e.g. 140 pounds of weight = 70 ounces of water)
- Limit other beverages to two cups per day of caffeine, and as a general practice, stay away from sugary beverages such as fruit juices and soda.
- Eighty to ninety percent of meals and snacks should come from organic, whole food sources.
- Maintain a diet of 60–70 percent non-starchy vegetables, 25 percent antibiotic-free and hormone-free protein, and approximately 5 percent gluten-free grains. Add in a small amount of low-glycemic fruit to your daily diet.

Two Years and Later following Delivery

Most women go through a normal healing process following childbirth. If complications occur, they can slow down your overall recovery well beyond two years. The risk of complications such as uterine, bladder or kidney infections, or postpartum depression, can be dramatically reduced by continuing with your nutritional plan to support optimal health status. As a guideline, try to stay within these dietary parameters:

- Sixty to seventy-five percent organic vegetables
- Twenty to thirty percent antibiotic-free andhormone-free protein sources
- Five percent low-glycemic fruit
- Five percent gluten-free grains
- No more than two cups of caffeine per day
- Avoid sugary beverages such as fruit juices and soda.
- Drink half your body weight in ounces each day of purified, distilled, or filtered water. (e.g. 140 pounds of weight = 70 ounces of water)

Postpartum Depression

Postpartum depression (PPD, also called postnatal depression) is a mood disorder that is believed to affect one in ten women within the first year after childbirth.[6] Although experts haven't figured out a definitive cause for PPD, there is strong speculation that it is due to fluctuating hormones during pregnancy.[7] These hormones (estrogen and progesterone) drop quickly after childbirth which results in chemical changes in the brain, triggering mood swings. More recent research also zeros in on sleep deprivation being a contributing factor.[8] Symptoms of PPD can vary, but some of the common symptoms are:

- Feeling overwhelmed or guilty
- Not bonding with the baby
- Being irritated, angry or moody
- Extreme sadness and hopelessness
- Lack of appetite

- Inability to sleep and/or concentrate
- Feeling disconnected from life or the rest of the world

Many people have heard the term "baby blues," which refers to a woman feeling "down" after delivering her baby. Postpartum depression is more severe and lasts longer. If left untreated, it can continue for many months and end up interfering with Mom's ability to properly care for her child, maintain her home, cook meals or hold down a job outside of the home.[9]

Research has also shown that many new moms with PPD have low serotonin or norepinephrine levels in the brain that are worsened by nutritional deficiencies. In many cases, particularly with low levels of norepinephrine, antidepressant drugs are little help with this kind of depression. Taking a look at possible nutritional deficiencies is recommended, particularly for women who are breastfeeding and want to avoid medications.

Specific Nutritional and Lifestyle Recommendations for Postpartum Depression

- Have your iron levels checked. Supplement if low.
- Take a B-complex vitamin daily.
- Increase your intake of good quality omega-3s (wild-caught salmon, sardines, anchovies, flaxseeds, chia seeds), or supplement with a high-quality fish oil such as krill or EPA/DHA combination.
- Herbal supplements can be very effective in treating depression or other mood disorders, but if you are still breastfeeding, check with your doctor or an herbalist first. Try St. John's Wort or Gingko Biloba,

following dosage instructions on the manufacturer's label. Either of these herbal supplements can be taken along with other nutritional supplements listed above.

- Make sure you stay properly hydrated every day. You should be drinking half your body weight in ounces of distilled, purified, or filtered water each day. (e.g. 140 pounds of weight = 70 ounces of water) Hydration is critical for proper blood volume, nutrient absorption, health of tissues and organs, and brain health.
- Avoid alcohol consumption.
- Use of recreational drugs is just dumb. You have a child who is dependent on you; don't even consider it.
- Find time to relax, rest whenever possible, and make time for an activity that calms you (reading, painting, or something else).
- Do deep breathing for three to five minutes at least once per day.
- Accept help from friends and family.
- Acknowledge how you're feeling, talk to close friends and family, consult your physician, and ask for help.

Breastfeeding: Nutritional Guidelines

Breastfeeding your newborn infant prolongs the exquisite miracle of childbirth. Many would say it is an opportunity to bond with your baby in a way that words can't describe. I found a few quotations below that help capture the essence of this remarkable experience.

> *"Breastfeeding is an unsentimental meta-phor for how love works, in a way. You don't decide how much and how deeply to love—*

*you respond to the beloved, and give with
joy exactly as much as they want."*

—*Marni Jackson*

"Breastfeeding is a gift that lasts a lifetime."

—*unknown author*

*"With his small head pillowed against your
breast and your milk warming his insides,
your baby knows a closeness to you. He is
gaining a firm foundation in an important
era of life—he is learning about love."*

—*unknown author*

Nursing your baby is truly an indescribable experience, one that inexplicably connects you, one with the other. Creating that bond may be your first motivation for choosing to breastfeed, but in reality, it provides benefits that stay with your baby for his or her entire life.

In the last twenty to thirty years, it has become common knowledge that breastfeeding is ideal for infant nutrition. Other benefits derived from nursing are also well known, such as the unique ability of the female body to prevent pregnancy while breastfeeding (although not 100 percent) and the protection of the infant from infection, disease, and malnutrition.

Breast milk is a complete food. Meaning: It naturally contains all the nutrients your baby needs for healthy, normal growth and development up to two years of age. Despite the remarkable ability a mother's milk has to nourish a newborn infant, the majority of women (over 80 percent), used man-ufactured formula from the early 1920s to the mid-1970s.[10] But in 1975 breastfeeding reclaimed its popularity and has since become widely known and accepted in the U.S. as the most beneficial way to nourish a newborn.[11] This renewed trend is due in large part to the efforts of our government agencies to educate young women, and medical professionals who advise them, about the benefits of breastfeeding to the infants and moms.[12]

I often disagree with the various dietary recommenda-tions coming from our so-called experts like the FDA, the USDA, or many of our traditional licensed healthcare pro-fessionals, but in this case, in my opinion, they are spot-on. There simply isn't a better option for nourishing your baby. Unless you have a physical abnormality that prevents your body from producing milk, I sincerely hope that your deci-sion will be to breastfeed, and to do so for as long as your lifestyle and schedule allows.

According to the CDC, the statistic of breastfeeding newborns was 81 percent as of 2013.[13] Between 40 and 50 percent of these women continued to breastfeed for three to six months, but only 22 percent did so exclusively (did not introduce other foods).[14] Although many doctors, midwives, lactation specialists, and even nutritionists will recommend breastfeeding for two years or longer, research shows us that even a minimum of three to six months provides critical nutrient support and protection to a newborn.[15]

In order to make your decision on this important topic, chances are you have been doing plenty of research on the pros and cons, health benefits to you and your baby, as well as the physical changes to expect prior to and during breast-feeding. There are so many terrific resources available to help you sort through those topics and educate yourself that I have decided in *Baby Maker* to focus your attention on two specific areas that you may gloss over, not understanding their importance.

The first is to really do some soul-searching on how you feel about breastfeeding. Why do I say that? Because your attitude, confidence, and knowledge about the health benefits will all play a role in whether you perceive breastfeeding to be healthier—easier and more convenient—or view it as an inconvenience—restrictive and uncomfortable. It isn't enough to be on the fence about breastfeeding during your pregnancy and think you're going to make a game-time decision when they hand you your baby in the delivery room. Yes, breastfeeding is a natural part of what a woman's body provides, but that does not mean you will instinctively know how to handle every nuance or issue that arises. As an example, if you know in advance that your newborn will need to nurse every one and a half to three hours during the first few weeks, you are less likely to worry that something is wrong when your baby cries to be fed that often.

Arming yourself with knowledge obtained from self-education, as well as consulting with experts, will help set you up with realistic goals and expectations. Being emotionally and mentally prepared will help build your confidence, shore up your commitment, and help set the stage for a positive, healthful experience.

The second important point I want to cover is for you to understand how vital your own health is prior to and during breastfeeding in order to ensure you are producing nutrient-dense milk for your baby.

The demands placed on a woman's body during the time it is producing milk are significant. If you have been following my nutritional strategy for pre-conception and pregnancy, then you can be assured you are well nourished and well equipped to produce milk packed with nutrients for your baby. Our goal now is to make sure you stay that way throughout the weeks or months your milk is the primary or exclusive source of nutrition for your little angel. If your nutritional or health status falters—if you go back to a high-sugar, high-carbohydrate, processed-food dietary plan—your body is likely to rebel by producing inadequate amounts of breast milk.

Nutritional requirements during breastfeeding, although similar to the requirements during pregnancy, are unique. Many women will continue taking their prenatal vitamin during lactation to support the nutritional demands, but this is not advisable. As an example, prenatal vitamins usually contain a higher amount of iron than is needed during breastfeeding. Continuing with the prenatal vitamin and the same dosage of iron after delivery is typically not needed. If you continue with the prenatal, you may find yourself dealing with constipation or other symptoms.

The other mindset that is common among new moms is to stop taking all supplements and rely on food sources for ongoing nutrition. This is also not advisable for nursing moms. In Chapter 9 I describe in detail the importance of taking supplements, especially when lab results show current nutrient levels are deficient, or demands for higher nutrient levels are being placed on the body, as in the case of pregnancy or nursing. Deficiencies or meeting unusual demands on the body are very difficult—if not impossible—to satisfy through food intake alone. By the time our food is harvested, packed, shipped, unpacked at your local food store, stored in your refrigerator, and eventually cooked, it has lost a large percentage of its nutrient value—up to 50 percent (in some cases even more). In addition to the minimal nutrients found in our food supply, it is extremely difficult to keep track of your food intake to ensure you are consuming the right amounts of everything you need. The use of nutritional supplements is key in restoring optimal health and nutrient levels. Switching to a postnatal vitamin or an appropriately formulated multivitamin immediately following delivery is the way to go for nursing moms.

Lactation puts fairly heavy demands on moms' nutrient levels. In some cases, these deficiencies will affect the content in her breast milk, which means your baby is at risk for the same deficiencies. In other cases the breast milk is protected from the deficiencies, leaving only the mother vulnerable to the effects those deficiencies can cause. My goal is to protect the health of you *and* your baby. To do that I would like to help you focus on maintaining proper levels of each nutrient that is vital to both of you following delivery.

In addition to the detailed chart that follows, I want to highlight five specific nutrients because these are often deficient following delivery.

Common Deficient Nutrients after Delivery Effecting Breastfeeding and Mom's Health

Calcium + Vitamin K2—Pregnancy and breastfeeding cause a temporary decrease in bone mass. This loss cannot be prevented by consuming additional calcium during pregnancy or while breastfeeding but usually returns to normal after breastfeeding has stopped. A daily minimum of 1200 mg of calcium along with 200 mcg of vitamin K2 (helps shuttle calcium to the bones) is required following delivery to support your body's efforts to regenerate proper bone mass.[16] Food sources for calcium include dairy products, yogurt, green vegetables, and bone broths.

Vitamin D—Absorption of calcium depends upon having an adequate level of vitamin D3. Breastfeeding women require an estimated 600 IUs per day.[17] Milk can be a good source of vitamin D3 but can also be very inflammatory. No more than one cup of milk is advisable. A supplement providing vitamin D3 alone, or calcium plus vitamin D3, is also a good source. (Check with your pediatrician to see whether your baby should also be given a vitamin D3 supplement. Breastmilk typically does not contain sufficient amounts of this important nutrient.)

Iron—It is advisable to have your iron levels checked following delivery. Women who are not anemic after delivery and who breastfeed exclusively seldom need an iron supplement. This is because they usually do not have a menstrual period for the first four to six months. Therefore, iron is not lost in menstrual blood. The recommended dietary allowance of iron for adult breastfeeding women is a minimum of 30 mg daily, compared with 18 mg for women who are not breastfeeding.[18] For breastfeeding women, prenatal vitamins contain higher amounts of iron, which are needed during pregnancy. However, these higher amounts can cause constipation if you continue to take it after delivery. If you develop problems with constipation, switch to a multivitamin that has a lower dose of iron or a no-iron formula.

Fish Oil—The American Academy of Pediatrics recommends that nursing mothers take in 200 to 300 mg of omega-3 fatty acids per day.[19] Women can meet this need with one to two servings of fish per week, such as herring, tuna, or salmon. To reduce exposure to mercury, moms should avoid predatory fish such as shark, swordfish, king mackerel, or tilefish, which can have high levels of mercury. (Visit www.edf.org for more details on how to choose fish free of toxins)

Nutrients Required during Breastfeeding[20]

(Dosages are given in a range of minimum to safe maximum.)

Nutrient	Daily Amount (min to safe maximum)	Food Sources
Calories	2,500–3,200	All food sources combined
Fiber	25–45 g	Beans, vegetables, gluten-free whole grains, nuts and seeds, berries. Best: raspberries, cauliflower, collard greens, broccoli, Swiss chard, spinach.
Protein	65–90 g	Fish, eggs, animal meats, vegetables, lentils. Best: cod, tuna, shrimp, venison, turkey, scallops, chicken, grass-fed beef, lamb, liver, spinach.

Fluids	Approximately 3 quarts or 96 ounces.	Purified, filtered, or distilled water; decaffeinated tea; unsweetened mineral water; organic whole milk; unsweetened almond or coconut milk.
Fish oil omega-3 fatty acids	200–300 mg	Most seafood, flaxseeds, walnuts, cauliflower, cabbage, romaine lettuce, broccoli, brussels sprouts, winter squash, summer squash, collard greens, spinach, kale, strawberries, green beans.
Vitamin A	7,000–10,000 IU	Carrots, spinach, kale, parsley, bell peppers, romaine lettuce, liver, Swiss chard, sweet potatoes, collard greens, cantaloupe, winter squash, apricots, broccoli, tomatoes, asparagus, green beans, brussels sprouts.
Vitamin D	400–600 IU	Shrimp, sardines, milk, cod, eggs

Vitamin E	60–400 IU	Sunflower seeds, Swiss chard, almonds, spinach, collard greens, kale, papaya, olives, bell peppers, brussels sprouts, kiwi, blueberries, tomatoes, broccoli.
Vitamin B1 (Thiamin)	1.6–25.0 mg	Romaine lettuce, asparagus, cremini mushrooms, spinach, sunflower seeds, tuna, green peas, tomatoes, eggplant, brussels sprouts, celery, cabbage, watermelon, bell peppers, carrots, summer squash, winter squash, green beans, broccoli, corn, kale, black beans, oats, pineapple.
Vitamin B2 (Riboflavin)	1.7–25.0 mg	Cremini mushrooms, liver, spinach, romaine lettuce, asparagus, Swiss chard, broccoli, collard greens, venison, yogurt, eggs, milk, green beans, celery, kale, cabbage, strawberries, tomatoes, cauliflower, raspberries, brussels sprouts, summer squash.

Vitamin B3 (Niacin)	18–100 mg	Cremini mushrooms, tuna, chicken, salmon, liver, asparagus, lamb, turkey, tomatoes, shrimp, sardines, summer squash, green peas, cod, collard greens, peanuts, carrots, broccoli, spinach, eggplant, cauliflower, grass-fed beef, raspberries, kale.
Vitamin B5 (Pantothenic acid)	7–250 mg	Cremini mushrooms, cauliflower, broccoli, liver, sunflower seeds, tomatoes, strawberries, yogurt, eggs, winter squash, collard greens, Swiss chard, corn.
Vitamin B6 (Pyridoxine)	10–100 mg	Spinach, bell peppers, garlic, tuna, cauliflower, bananas, broccoli, celery, asparagus, cabbage, cremini mushrooms, kale, collard greens, brussels sprouts, watermelon, cod, Swiss chard, tomatoes, carrots, summer squash, eggplant.

Vitamin B12 (Cobalamin)	25–500 mcg	Liver, sardines, venison, shrimp, scallops, salmon, grass-fed beef, lamb, cod, yogurt, milk, eggs.
Vitamin B9 (Folate or 5-MTHFR)	400–800 mcg	Romaine lettuce, spinach, asparagus, liver, collard greens, broccoli, cauliflower, beets, lentils, celery, brussels sprouts, beans, summer squash, cabbage, green peas.
Biotin	200–500 mcg	Peanuts, almonds, Swiss chard, goat's milk, yogurt, tomatoes, eggs, carrots, onions, avocados, milk, walnuts, salmon, cashews, sesame seeds, bananas.
Choline	100–250 mg	Shrimp, eggs, scallops, chicken, turkey, tuna, cod, salmon, grass-fed beef, collard greens.
Inositol	100–250 mg	Beans, whole grains, cantaloupe, citrus fruits (except lemon)

Vitamin C	120–2,000 mg	Bell peppers, parsley, broccoli, strawberries, cauliflower, lemon juice, romaine lettuce, brussels sprouts, papaya, kale, kiwi, cantaloupe, oranges, grapefruit, cabbage, tomatoes, Swiss chard, collard greens, raspberries, asparagus, celery, spinach, pineapple, green beans.
Bioflavonoids	125–250 mg	Most fruits and vegetables.
Calcium + vitamin K2	Calcium 1,200–1,600 mg Vitamin K2 200 mcg	Spinach, collard greens, basil, cinnamon, yogurt, Swiss chard, cheese, kale, milk, goat's milk, rosemary, romaine lettuce, celery, sesame seeds, broccoli, cabbage, green beans, summer squash, garlic, mustard seeds, brussels sprouts, asparagus.
Chloride	2–4 g	Salt, sea salt, seaweed, rye, tomatoes, lettuce, celery, olives.
Chromium	50–400 mcg	Romaine lettuce, onions, tomatoes

Copper	2–3 mg	Liver, cremini mushrooms, Swiss chad, spinach, sesame seeds, kale, summer squash, asparagus, eggplant, cashews, tomatoes, sunflower seeds, ginger, green beans, potatoes, sweet potatoes, kiwi, pumpkin seeds, lentils, walnuts.
Iodine	290–400 mcg	Sea vegetables (arame, nori, kombu, hijiki, miso), yogurt, milk, eggs, strawberries.
Iron	30–50 mg	Spinach, Swiss chard, basil, romaine lettuce, shiitake mushrooms, green beans, parsley, kale, shrimp, broccoli, brussels sprouts, asparagus, olives, lentils, venison, pumpkin seeds, sesame seeds, celery, quinoa.

Magnesium	450–1,000 mg	Swiss chard, spinach, summer squash, pumpkin seeds, broccoli, basil, cucumbers, flaxseeds, green beans, celery, collard greens, kale, mustard seeds, sunflower seeds, ginger, quinoa, salmon, black beans, beets, tomatoes, cremini mushrooms.
Manganese	2.5–15 mg	Cinnamon, romaine lettuce, pineapple, spinach, collard greens, raspberries, Swiss chard, kale, garlic, grapes, summer squash, strawberries, oats, green beans, brown rice, broccoli, beets, flaxseeds, cremini mushrooms, cauliflower.
Molybdenum	150–250 mcg	Beans, lentils, grains.
Phosphorus	1,200–1,600 mg	Milk, meats, beans, lentils, nuts, whole grains, vegetables.

Potassium	2–5 g	Swiss chard, cremini mushrooms, spinach, romaine lettuce, celery, broccoli, winter squash, tomatoes, collard greens, summer squash, eggplant, cantaloupe, green beans, brussels sprouts, kale, carrots, beets, papaya, asparagus, basil, cucumbers, cauliflower.
Selenium	150–300 mcg	Cremini mushrooms, cod, shiitake mushrooms, shrimp, tuna, liver, sardines, salmon, mustard seeds, eggs, turkey, lamb, oats, chicken, grass-fed beef, sunflower seeds, garlic, broccoli, asparagus.
Zinc	25–40 mg	Liver, cremini mushrooms, spinach, grass-fed beef, lamb, summer squash, asparagus, venison, chard, shrimp, collard greens, pumpkin seeds, yogurt, green peas, broccoli, sesame seeds.

The Formula-Fed Infant

As mentioned earlier, a large percentage of women having children in the U.S. are breastfeeding, and doing so for a minimum of three months. However, in 2012 a study was published in the journal *Pediatrics* that stated of the moms who plan to breastfeed exclusively for three months or longer, less than one-third of them actually achieve this goal.[21] While it is not my intention to put anyone on a guilt trip, I want to encourage these women to reconsider before making a final decision not to breastfeed or to discontinue it too soon in your infant's development.

There are cases where a woman may have physical limitations that make breastfeeding challenging or even impossible. Also common are those who attempt to breast feed but struggle with adequate milk production or do not receive adequate support from hospital staff where delivery occurred.

More than 85 percent of women in the U.S. who enter a hospital to deliver have an intention of breastfeeding exclusively, but only about one-third of these moms actually meet this goal.[22] According to research, three-quarters of all U.S. hospitals end up supplementing with formula during the time an infant is in their care.[23] I can personally relate to these statistics. I was one of the many women who was steadfast in my decision to breastfeed only to have it all fall apart when my milk production was not adequate. After giving birth (both times), the nursing staff was giving my baby formula in between breastfeeding sessions. Although I'm sure these healthcare providers are well intended, such practices are associated with delayed onset of adequate milk production and premature abandonment of breastfeeding by the new mom.

Whatever the reasons, choosing to bottle feed with infant formula is a personal decision and one that should be made after considerable research and thought. Women who want to breastfeed should seek guidance, education, and ongoing support from knowledgeable providers who can help and advise them. Make sure you communicate clearly your preferences for feeding your newborn to your obstetrician, pediatrician, and hospital support staff.

La Leche League International, www.llli.org/webus.html, is an excellent resource for women whose goal it is to exclusively breastfeed and would like expert guidance and support.

Sleep-Deprivation

After nine months of growing a baby inside you, and countless hours of labor and delivery, you shouldn't be surprised to learn that most women will describe feeling completely exhausted or "wiped out." Of course, it varies from one woman to the next, but the need for rest, relaxation, and sleep right after delivering is common.

Years ago it was normal for hospitals to keep a new mom and baby for two or three nights in the hospital, which gave everyone (Mom and Dad) a chance to get some much-needed sleep while their newborn was being cared for by the nursing staff (except for the breastfeeding, of course!). Today, most health insurers only cover expenses for the first forty-eight hours (one night) after an "uncomplicated" vaginal delivery, or ninety-six hours for a C-section birth. It would probably be less time than that by now if our Congress hadn't stepped in back in 1996 and created the Newborns' and Mothers' Health Protection Act that requires insurance companies to cover the expenses of this minimal hospital stay.[24]

The point here is you will be tired after your precious little bundle arrives. Unless you make plans ahead of time to have help in your household, arrange for a longer stay in the hospital, or arrange for your spouse to have co-parent maternity leave, it will be challenging the first few days or weeks after getting home with your newborn.

Most new moms will agree that dealing with sleep-deprivation when you get your baby home is one of the most difficult adjustments to make. The tendency is for women to soldier through and just deal with it. But similar to postpartum depression, trying to cope with too little sleep is risky and can lead to other health problems.

According to a sleep study performed on postpartum women in 2005–06, sleep deprivation can develop into chronic insomnia, daytime sleepiness, cognitive deficits, fatigue, hormone imbalance, irritability, or other mood disorders, and it is directly correlated to postpartum depression.[25] A further complication of not getting enough sleep is the affect it can have on the quantity of milk being produced in a breastfeeding mom.

Below are a few tips to help you cope with tiredness and sleep-deprivation:

- Rest whenever you can. It doesn't matter if you have visitors or the dirty dishes are piled high in the kitchen sink; if you have an opportunity to lie down and close your eyes for even a few minutes, do it.
- Sleep when your baby sleeps. Most newborns do a lot of sleeping in between their nursing schedule. Take advantage of their sleep schedule.
- Make sure you're staying hydrated with plenty of purified, filtered, or distilled water. Proper hydration

levels help nutrients from your food get absorbed and transported efficiently, help blood-flow, support your kidneys and bladder in filtering out waste and toxins, help you fight fatigue by maintaining healthy cellular activity, help regulate blood pressure, and provide other benefits. While breastfeeding, your body needs around ninety-six ounces of healthy, unsweetened, decaffeinated fluids per day.

- Maintain a healthy diet of organic, fresh whole foods. Now is not the time to start filling up on caffeine, sweets, or other junk food to save yourself time or to get that quick boost of energy. Right now, your body is deficient of several key nutrients from bringing your baby into the world and is desperate for nutrient-dense foods to replenish itself. A whole-foods diet is the fastest way to restore your energy levels, hormone balance, and overall health status.

- Call friends and family for help. Don't be afraid to ask for help with household chores, meal preparation, running errands, or even taking a turn at caring for your baby for a couple of hours (or an afternoon). If you don't have friends and family who can be available, consider hiring a postpartum doula for your first week or two at home. They are women who are experienced in "mothering," caring for newborns, and often are willing to help with housework, cooking, or caring for other children in your home.

- Don't invite people to stay in your home with you after your baby arrives unless it is someone who can respect your privacy boundaries, truly wants to help you around the house, and is someone who is pleasant to be around. Even the most well-intended houseguest will become a burden if it is someone who raises your stress levels or isn't willing to help you out in the manner you need.

- If you work outside the home and are on maternity leave, do not check your email, voicemail messages, or respond to phone calls from your boss or co-workers who "just need a few quick moments of your time"—unless of course they are calling to congratulate you on your new arrival. Keep your communication all baby talk, not work-talk.

- Communicate your need for rest and sleep to your partner and family members. Take turns caring for your baby while the other person sleeps.

- Remind yourself often that everything you're going through is normal for a woman who just had a baby. Have realistic expectations for yourself that take into account the enormous amount of healing that is underway inside you. Be gentle with yourself.

- Treasure every moment and nuance of this newborn stage with your baby. At times it will seem never-ending because you are tired, depleted, and still in a healing phase, but in reality, the first few weeks go by in a blink as do all the "firsts" that your baby will have. You won't want to miss a single one of them!

- Remind yourself that the sleeplessness will eventually pass. Your baby will develop more consistent sleeping patterns over time, which will allow you to return to more normal patterns as well. Have patience. The challenging, difficult phases with infants are just that—phases—gradual changes in development that often disappear as quietly and quickly as they began.

CHAPTER 9

Not All Supplements Are Created Equal: Choose and Buy Supplements like a Pro

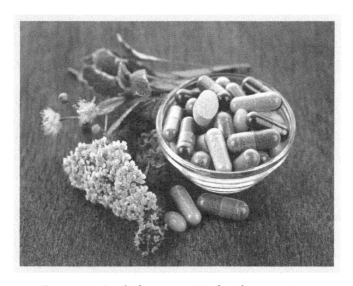

Source: BigStockPhoto.com. Used with permission.

Why Take Supplements?

There are practical, therapeutic reasons for taking supplements, and you should have at least a general idea of what they are. Don't rely exclusively on your healthcare practitioner or nutritionist. I always encourage my clients to get involved in their healthcare decisions and educate themselves on the significance of various decisions pertaining to their care. Don't bury your head in the sand when it comes to what you're putting into your body, whether that is food or supplements.

In many respects, supplements are no different than food—quality makes a difference.

The Centers for Disease Control and Prevention tells us that as of 2006, over half of the adults in the U.S. use dietary supplements, mostly multivitamins (39 percent).[1] Despite this trend, it does not seem to be making people healthier since chronic disease rates continue to rise. And herein lies the important point with supplements: Supplements must be used *in addition to a healthy diet*, not in place of one.

You can't cover up years of abuse to your body from processed foods, a high-sugar diet, frequent fast foods, smoking, or excessive alcohol use by simply taking a handful of pills every day. Many Americans try that route every day with pharmaceutical drugs and usually figure out that, in most cases, they only mask symptoms and often with terrible side-affects that can be worse than the original problem.

It's likely that a large number of those people who use supplements are not noticing any health benefits at all, which explains why you can ask ten different people for their opinion on taking supplements and get several different responses.

The confusion shows up among pregnant women as well.

It is fairly common for obstetricians to recommend a prenatal vitamin if a woman is trying to conceive or is already pregnant. But yet only 13 percent of pregnant women actually take them.[2] This is very troubling for reasons you will understand as we get further into this topic.

When the CDC checked this out with a survey, they got somewhat better results—33 percent of women of childbearing age reported taking their supplements, but a much larger group, 84 percent, acknowledged awareness of the benefits associated with them.[3] So the vast majority of women understand that supplements offer health benefits during pregnancy, but only a third of them can actually be bothered to take them? Meanwhile, there is documented proof that a large number (50 to 70 percent) of serious infant health conditions such as neural tube defects could be avoided by taking a folic acid   supplement a few months prior to conception.[4] I recommend the natural form called folate, which is one of the B vitamins. Folic acid is a synthetic version of folate that is difficult for the body to breakdown and utilize, and there is evidence to suggest it increases the chance of cancer.[5]

What's going on here? We have the scientific knowledge and access to remedies that will help improve fertility, increase chances of a healthy baby and mom during pregnancy, and improve chances of preventing birth defects, and eager young soon-to-be moms aren't paying attention or taking it seriously. Interesting.

In the CDC report, the pitiful reasons given for not taking a vitamin or mineral supplement were:

- Forgetting (28 percent)
- Didn't think they needed them (16 percent)

- Believing they got enough nutrients from their diet (9 percent)

Now you know why I decided to write this book. Clearly, more education is needed among women and men of child-bearing age.[6]

Everyone Is Nutrient-Deficient

I believe in taking supplements and they are a regular part of my recommendations to clients in my nutrition counseling practice. But let me be clear: As I stated before, they cannot make up for an unhealthy lifestyle. Doctor Mercola stated this best:

> *"It has always been my belief and teaching that supplements are in addition to not in place of a good sound diet. You can't cover your nutritional or lifestyle "sins" by taking a handful of supplements. Biology doesn't work that way."*

> —*Doctor Joseph Mercola, 2011*

If you thoroughly read this book and take its recommendations and principles to heart, you will be clear about the fact that nutritious whole foods come first, lifestyle decisions a very close second, and supplements third, but—during pregnancy especially—it is the aggregate of all three that creates a powerhouse of health benefits.

Is Your Food "Healthy"?

First you need to understand that in today's world it is challenging, if not nearly impossible, to provide our bodies with the nutrients it needs on a daily basis using food as your only source of those nutrients. If you are like most people living in the U.S., a large part of your diet includes fast-food restaurants, processed and refined foods, and beverages and foods that are high in sugar. You'll know this is true by taking note of the average size person you see as you sit in your parked car at your local grocery store. More than one-third of adults in the U.S. are obese and 10 percent diagnosed with type 2 diabetes.[7]

Even if you are one of the few who manage to avoid those dietary pitfalls and focus on fresh, whole foods as the staples in your daily diet, the fruits and vegetables you consume are most often grown and harvested from nutrient-depleted soil. The meats are from livestock that are raised on chemically modified grains and hormones. The food you and I consume every day, by and large, is deficient in nutrients and loaded with harmful chemicals, fats, and calories that contribute to the various health epidemics we witness in this country.

The food supply available to us in the U.S. has been compromised and no longer offers the amount of nutrients our ancestors consumed by eating the same foods a century ago. In fact, a 2004 study done by the University of Texas showed since the 1930s we have seen a 15 percent decline in nutrients in fruits and vegetables and a 30 to 50 percent decline in the protein content in wheat and barley.[8] This doesn't take into account the additional nutrients lost from the use of pesticides and herbicides, what is lost naturally after a crop is harvested, or during packaging and shipping to your local area. In most cases, additional nutrients are also lost once you get your food home and cook it.

So the sad and unfortunate fact is that you can be as dedicated to an organic, fresh, whole foods diet as Weston A. Price (known as the "Isaac Newton of Nutrition"), but your body could still be deficient in important nutrients.[9]

All of these facts, in my opinion, make a strong case for incorporating nutritional supplements into your dietary and lifestyle routine.

On the following pages I will explain in detail what supplements you should be taking to support conception and pregnancy and why. I will also give you information on how to purchase high-quality supplements and why quality is important, as well as a few suggestions on where to shop for supplements.

If you are at a stage where you are thinking of getting pregnant, please refer to my "Conception Strategy" for men and women in Chapter 2. Ideally, you will be at least six to eight months in advance of your anticipated conception date, which means now is the perfect time to start your prenatal and/or supplement regimen.

For those of you who are already pregnant or have already delivered your precious little baby—as I said in Chapter 3—don't panic. It's never too late to work on getting healthy! You and your baby are well worth the effort no matter when you get started.

Who Is Paying Attention to Supplement Manufacturers?

As it turns out, a lot of people! All those little bottles of tablets and capsules you see in your stores and online are part of an exploding industry. In the U.S. it is expected to reach 278 billion dollars by 2024.[10] You can imagine the attention it is getting. Everyone who is remotely connected to healthcare is trying to get a piece of this lucrative industry. And with that kind of growth potential comes plenty of competition that runs the entire spectrum between high quality and junk. Consumers need to be informed when choosing supplements.

The pharmaceutical companies would love for you to believe that a prescription-grade prenatal vitamin is your only safe option, even though they are considerably more expensive than over-the-counter products, unless you have insurance.

You will also find plenty of disparaging information in the media about over-the-counter supplements. (Can you guess who is behind most of it?) With all this nastiness surrounding supplements, it would be easy to conclude that the dietary supplement industry is a "free-for-all," with no regulations or oversight whatsoever, but that couldn't be further from the truth.

While the scrutiny and regulations are vastly more intense for pharmaceutical drugs—and they should be given the often-devastating side-affects that go along with many of them—the FDA has created a means by which the consumer can identify high-quality dietary supplements.

There is a great deal of information available for people who really want to learn how to identify quality supplements. If you're the bookworm type and want to become a guru in supplements, you will study up on a few areas: the types of inert substances that are used to achieve a specific consistency (i.e., tablet versus capsule), the types of binders, fillers, or lubricants that are used, whether the nutrients used are natural or synthetic, and how many ingredients are used that are known allergens such as wheat, corn, milk, yeast, and artificial coloring.

There is a similar amount of information on the manufacturing process, not to mention the rules and regulations that apply to this fast-growing industry. Most of this detail is way out of scope for this book, so if you are pregnant or planning to be and just want to know what you should be taking and how to pick good ones, I am going to summarize it all down to a few key points you need to know.

Don't Waste Your Money—Buy Quality

Step #1—Choosing Quality Supplements—Watch for the GMP Label

One of the first things you can do is also one of the most important. When choosing supplements, look for the GMP label. It is called the Good Manufacturing Practice (sometimes referred to as cGMP or Current Good Manufacturing Practice). The rule for GMP was published in 2007 and reads as follows:

> *"The Dietary Supplement cGMP rule requires persons who manufacture, package, label or hold a dietary supplement to establish and follow current good manufacturing practice to ensure the quality of the dietary supplement and to ensure that the dietary supplement is packaged and labeled as specified in the master manufacturing record."*[1]

This is important for safety reasons. You want to make sure that the supplement contains only those ingredients and substances listed on the label. We've all heard some of the horror stories in the media about supplements that were found to contain rogue ingredients. Purchasing only GMP-labeled products eliminates this concern.

There is another, more stringent oversight program I will briefly mention. It is called the "Natural Products Association" or NPA and has been around since 1936, long before the FDA officially launched GMP. Although it has undergone several name changes over the decades, NPA is "the oldest nonprofit association dedicated to serving and preserving the rights of natural product industry retailers and suppliers."[12] The NPA oversees their TruLabel program, which is a testing program for supplement suppliers to ensure products meet the claims made on their labels. Their certification program for supplement manufacturers is called the "NPA GMP" and administers minimum standards to ensure dietary supplements are manufactured consistently with respect to purity of ingredients, potency, and composition.[13] In short, they make sure a supplement contains the ingredients it claims to contain.

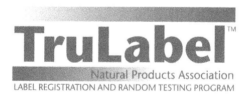

Source: Natural Products Association, www. npainfo.org. Used with permission.

Here's the bottom line: good quality supplements taken according to instructions are safe. According to Orthomolecular.org in 2005:

"Over a 27-year period, vitamin supplements have been alleged to have caused the deaths

of a total of eleven people in the U.S. A new analysis of U.S. Poison Control Center annual report data indicates that there have, in fact, been no deaths whatsoever from vitamins.... none at all, in the 27 years that such reports have been available.[14]

The manufacturing and labeling process is monitored. If a supplement maker does not meet their criteria for certification, either they will not be approved or their existing certification will be revoked. Neither the FDA or NPA is shy about pulling a product from distribution or completely shutting down a facility's operation. In fact, according to Doctor Mercola, the FDA has ramped up their auditing efforts recently and is hot on the trail of offenders.[15] These agencies and others have full authority under current regulations to do whatever they have to do to ensure consumer and product safety.

Invest a little time to identify high-quality supplements for yourself. Provided you follow the dosage recommendations and other instructions from your healthcare provider, you can scratch "safety" off your list of things to worry about. If you don't trust your own abilities and knowledge to make your own selections, contact a knowledgeable healthcare practitioner for help.

Step #2—Choosing Quality Supplements— Buy "Quality," Not Price

Buying "quality" supplements does not necessarily mean more expensive. Even inferior products can be over-priced. Similar to selecting food, it is important to review product labels and know at least the key basic facts about supplements.

As outlined above, the first step in buying quality supplements is to look for the GMP label. Other important criteria include the categories below along with a brief description of each one.

Does the supplement contain natural or synthetic nutrients?

Choose natural whenever possible. I used to think all supplements were synthetic since they are manufactured. After all, you can't grow and harvest a vitamin B-complex capsule out of the ground, so it can't be "natural," right? Nope! There actually is a difference between natural and synthetic nutrients.

From a chemist's standpoint, their molecular structure is the same, but where they differ is in how the elements or atoms are arranged.[16] Synthesized nutrients are mirror images of their natural counterparts, and it is a difference the human body can recognize. For instance, the natural version of vitamin E is three times more absorbable than its synthetic mirror image.[17] Also, naturally sourced nutrients will often contain additional co-factors—enzymes and phytonutrients (plant-based nutrients), which have a synergistic effect on the overall performance of the supplement. So whenever you have a choice between natural versus synthetic, go with the natural formula as the better choice.

Does the supplement claim to contain nutrients that are food-grown, food-based, or whole-food concentrates?

The best choice is whole-food concentrates. Just because a label uses the word "food" does not mean it is completely natural. You will often see "food-based" on a supplement label when purified synthetic vitamins are added to a "base" of food such as herbs, spirulina, or wheat grass.[18]

"Food-grown" or "food-formed" supplements are made by introducing synthetic vitamins into inorganic minerals to a base of living yeast. Through fermentation the yeast takes in the nutrients, which then become part of the living food. Nutrients made this way are not necessarily harmful. Some manufacturers claim this process may increase absorption. What we do know is they often have lower potencies and can be a problem for people suffering from allergies, especially those who have issues with candida.[19]

The "whole-food concentrates" are nutrients that are created by freeze-drying vegetables, green foods, and other whole foods that captures and preserves all the nutrients and co-factors in the food. This process retains the original structure of the nutrient, nutrient ratios, and potency.

Is the packaging sufficient to preserve potency?

The supplements you select should be packaged in a tightly sealed, opaque or dark-colored container that protects the supplement inside it from light, heat, or moisture. Most nutrients will lose their potency and purity much faster if exposed to air, heat, contaminants, light, or moisture. It is equally important for you to store your supplements properly once you have them home. Many supplements will be labeled with storage recommendations such as "do not expose to heat," "store in cool, dry location," or "best if refrigerated." Again, read the labels and always follow the instructions provided.

Does the packaging contain ingredient details?

The best manufacturers will provide you with as much information about the ingredients contained in their product as physically possible with the space limitations on the label.

Stay away from supplement brands that can't be bothered to provide milligram amounts and a complete description about the form of the nutrient. Does it just say "calcium" or the more complete description "calcium citrate" or "calcium carbonate"? Does it clearly list the amount of each ingredient?

There are many other areas that can be explored if you really wanted to become your own nutritional supplement expert. Those listed above are the ones I believe to be the most important. Using them as guidelines will help you get the most health benefit from those you purchase and use.

Where to Buy Supplements

I have listed a few of my favorite websites and supplement brands in this section. If you are working with an infertility specialist or gynecologist/obstetrician, they often will prescribe a prescription-grade vitamin for you. No matter where you purchase your prenatal multi from, you should look closely at the nutrient levels contained in it. If there are deficiencies from the recommended levels here, you should manage your food intake and additional supplements to fill in where necessary.

The internet has become a great marketplace for nutritional supplements just as it has for many other items we purchase regularly. Many of my clients will simply search for a supplement brand I give them and purchase it on Amazon, but there are also wholesale distributors with whom many practitioners are registered and allowed to offer discounts to their clients.

Hopefully, at this point you understand that where you purchase *from* is not as important as *what* you purchase. Most brick-and-mortar stores will offer a diverse selection of supplement brands. And of course there are plenty of online

22

sources, some even low-cost, but be careful—the quality supplements will usually be offered alongside poorer-quality brands. Reading labels and having some basic knowledge about what you're looking for is important.

Online Websites for Purchasing Supplements

Amazon.com	Use search bar for specific brand names
Vitacost.com	Carries wide variety of brands, often at discount prices; check labels for quality
EmersonEcologics.com*	Access and discounts granted with permission from practitioner
Natural Partners.com*	Access and discounts granted with permission from practitioner
NutritionExpress.com	Carries wide variety of brands, check labels for quality
ThriveMarket.com*	Organic and non-GMO food brands

*Maintains high quality product standards

Following these guidelines will ensure that you use your money and time wisely when it comes to selecting nutritional supplements. Doing so requires you to start reading labels and doing a little homework to make sure dosages are sufficient, but the payoff will be virile fertility and a dramatically improved health status to support the beautiful life growing inside you.

APPENDIX

Bone Broth Recipe

What's in Bones That Makes Bone Broth So Good for You?

The health benefits of broth made with bones have been researched and documented for hundreds of years.

There are many nutritional benefits to consuming bone broth during your pre-conception planning and/or during pregnancy. There are three main components to this broth: gelatin (collagen), cartilage, and bone marrow—all incredibly important in supporting the development of connective tissue, cartilage, and bone. This nutrient-dense broth is also loaded with amino acids (building blocks of protein), minerals (calcium, magnesium, and phosphorus), and glucosamine and chondroitin to support mom's joints as her baby grows. In addition to its nutrient value, bone broth is a nourishing substitute during those times when nausea makes it difficult to eat and digest food during pregnancy. It is soothing to the stomach.

Choosing Bones for Bone Broth

You can purchase raw bones from a butcher or use bones left-over from cooking. For example, if you make a bone-in roast, save the bone(s) to make bone broth. If you cook a chicken, save the carcass. If you don't want to make broth right away (or you don't have enough bones), simply place the bones in a sealed freezer bag and store in the freezer until you're ready. When it's time to make broth, there's no need to defrost. Just toss the frozen bones right into the pot.

When purchasing bones for making homemade bone broth, aim for a variety of bone types, which will ensure you're getting marrow, cartilage, and gelatin in your broth. If you're adventurous, you can try adding a couple of (well-cleaned) chicken feet, which are an excellent source of collagen, along with the bones. For making beef or lamb bone broth, be sure to ask your butcher for both a joint bone and marrow bones.

Your number-one consideration when making bone broth is the quality of the bones you use. Do your best to source the highest quality bones possible from pasture-raised/free-range, grass-fed animals that have not been subjected to antibiotics and growth hormones.

How to Make Bone Broth

Some people prefer roasting the bones before making the broth this method as they find it adds extra flavor to the finished broth. Roasting is totally a taste preference and is not required. In any case, it is only for beef, lamb, or wild game bones—it is not a necessary step for bone broth made with poultry or fish.

If you do wish to roast the bones first, all you need to do is place the bones on a cookie sheet and roast uncovered in a 350°F oven for 20–30 minutes. Once you've gathered your bones (either raw or roasted), you're ready to proceed with the steps below.

Step #1: Place bones (fresh, frozen, or roasted) into a large stock pot or slow cooker and cover with cold filtered water. Make sure all the bones are covered, but still leave plenty of room for water to boil. Add coarsely chopped onion, carrots, and celery stalks to the pot.

Step #2: Add two tablespoons of an acidic substance (e.g., apple cider vinegar, wine, or lemon juice) to the water prior to cooking. The acid will help draw out important nutrients from the bones.

Step #3: Heat slowly, gradually bringing to a boil and then reduce heat to a simmer. Skim off any scum that floats to the top.

Step #4: Cook long and slow. Cook chicken bones for 6 to 48 hours. Beef bones can cook for 12 to 72 hours. A long and slow cooking time is necessary to fully extract the nutrients in and around the bones. You may need to add additional hot water as the broth simmers to keep the bones covered.

Step #5: Add additional vegetables and/or seasonings such as sea salt, pepper, herbs, and peeled garlic cloves to the pot 1–2 hours before finishing. Optionally, add a bunch of fresh parsley 10–15 minutes before removing from heat.

Step #6: Once broth is ready, remove from heat and allow broth to cool enough so you can handle the pot. Remove the solids, strain through a fine mesh strainer, and reserve the broth. If there had been meat on the bones, you can pick this out to use in a soup.

Step #7: Consume broth within 5–7 days or freeze for later use. Bone broth can be safely frozen for several months.

Bone Broth Tips

- Use a slow cooker that can be continually reset for several hours at a time. If using the stovetop, be sure to keep an eye on your broth and follow good stove safety practices.
- After the broth cools, a protective layer of fat will harden on top. Only discard this layer when you are about to eat the broth. Alternatively, you may choose to consume it along with the broth. If your bones are from quality pastured animals, this is a healthy, nutrient-dense source of fat.
- If your broth becomes thick and jelly-like—congratulations! That means it contains a significant amount of gelatin (collagen). When you heat up your broth, it will turn back into liquid form.
- To warm up your broth, scoop some into a saucepan and gently heat your broth on the stove, not in a microwave oven. This will retain the maximum nutrition. Season with salt and pepper and/or add other health-promoting spices such as turmeric, ginger, and so forth.
- There are many ways to use bone broth. It is delicious to drink by itself, or you can use it as a soup base, in sauces, or to replace the water when cooking rice, quinoa, or other grains.

Food Sources of Potassium

Food	Serving Size	Amount of Potassium (mg)
Swiss chard	1 cup	960.8
Cremini mushrooms	5 ounces	635.0
Spinach	1 cup	838.8
Romaine lettuce	2 cups	324.8
Celery	1 cup	344.4
Broccoli	1 cup	505.4
Winter squash	1 cup	895.9
Tomatoes	1 cup	399.6
Collard greens	1 cup	494.0
Summer squash	1 cup	345.6
Eggplant	1 cup	245.5
Cantaloupe	1 cup	494.4
Green beans	1 cup	373.8
Brussels sprouts	1 cup	494.5
Kale	1 cup	296.4
Carrots	1 cup	394.1
Beets	1 cup	518.5

Source: Mateljan, G. (2007). *The World's Healthiest Foods*. Seattle, WA: GMF Publishing[2]

Baby-Maker Fertility and Pregnancy Smoothie

Note: You must use a high-powered blender, such as a Vitamix or Nutribullet, that will liquefy fruits and vegetables to get a smooth, refined, "drinkable" consistency. It is not advisable to use a "juicer" that extracts only the liquids from fruits and vegetables. The remaining liquid from that process is highly concentrated in sugars.

Vegetable smoothies are an excellent way to increase your intake of vegetables. Smoothies or juicing should not replace eating and chewing solid foods at every meal, but they are a perfect meal alternative for busy working professionals or for anyone who doesn't have the inclination to sit down and eat the amount of vegetables every day that your body needs to support fertility or pregnancy.

I like to make a large quantity in advance so I, or anyone in my household, has a glass readily available throughout the day. A minimal amount of nutrient value will be lost when storing and refrigerating for a few hours, but for me it is worth the convenience of having them prepared in advance.

- This recipe makes about three 8-ounce servings.
- Use fresh, organic ingredients.
- Rinse all vegetables well before adding to blender.
- Use all parts of the stalk, leaf, and stems to maximize nutrient value.
- Lightly steam leafy greens before blending to minimize goitrogen content.
- If adding fruit, choose organic, low-glycemic fruit

Ingredients:

Purified or distilled water
2–3 cups (or substitute with brewed green tea)
Green or red kale stalks
1–3 stalks
Green or red Swiss chard
1–2 stalks
Collard greens
1–2 stalks
Dandelion greens
4–5 stems
Parsley
small bunch, approximately 3–4 stems
Eggs
(raw organic) 2–3
Avocado
⅓
Coconut oil
2 Tbsps.
Lemon
½ to 1 lemon (to taste), cut off ends only—the rest goes
    in the blender (rind too!). Lemon helps minimize
    bitterness from the veggies and is good for digestion.
Berries*
small handful (about 4–6 berries, little more
    if raspberries or blueberries)
Banana*
⅓ of banana, outer skin removed (eliminate if using
    berries or reduce quantities if using both fruits).
Optional ingredients:
Organic, brown-rice vanilla protein powder

½ scoop
NanoGreens or other powdered vegetable drink
½ scoop
Vitamin C powder
1 dose/scoop

Experiment with other vegetables such as broccoli, carrots, beets, other leafy greens, other herbal teas as a substitute for water (no fruit juice!), or boost protein and good quality fats by adding nuts and seeds such as flax, hemp, pumpkin, almonds, and walnuts.

Note: Women who are pregnant or breastfeeding should not be on a detoxification plan or using vegetable juices as their primary source of nourishment.

Summary of Foods to Avoid during Pregnancy

The following list of foods to avoid during pregnancy does not take into consideration other pre-existing health conditions that may require a stricter food elimination plan.

<u>Animal Protein</u>

- Bacon (except turkey bacon without nitrates and hormones; choose gluten-free
- Hot dogs (except chicken and turkey hot dogs without nitrates and hormones; choose gluten-free
- Tuna (all types—toro, albacore, ahi, and so forth, including canned)

<u>Grains</u>

- Barley
- Breads (unless gluten-free, sugar-free)
- Cereals (except gluten- and sugar-free varieties)
- Crackers (unless gluten- and sugar-free)
- Farro
- Kamut
- Oats (gluten-free okay)
- Pasta (unless made from brown rice, buckwheat, or quinoa)
- Pastries
- Rye
- Spelt
- Triticale
- White flours
- White rice
- Wheat (refined)
- Whole wheat

Vegetables

- Corn
- Mushrooms
- Potatoes (or eat sparingly, two or three servings per week)
- Beans and legumes (small amounts only, three or four servings per week, soak overnight before eating)

Nuts and Seeds

- Cashews
- Peanuts, peanut butter

Oils

- Canola oil
- Corn oil
- Cottonseed oil
- Peanut oil
- Processed oils and partially hydrogenated or fully hydrogenated oils
- Soy oil

Dairy*

- Cheeses (unless aged or organic—eat in small quantities only, three or four servings per week)
- Buttermilk
- Cow's milk
- Ice cream (infrequently for snacks only)
- Margarine
- Sour cream

- Yogurt (unless organic or from grass-fed sources—
  choose brands with fewer than 10 g of sugar and consume infrequently, three or four servings per week)

*Note: pregnant and nursing women should not consume
raw dairy products.

Fruits

The following fruits are high on the glycemic index and
therefore should be consumed infrequently and in small
quantities, two or three servings week.

- Apricots
- Bananas
- Cherries
- Cranberries (sweetened)
- Dried Fruits (including dates, figs, raisins, prunes)
- Guavas
- Grapes
- Juices (all, sweetened and unsweetened)
- Kiwis
- Mangoes
- Melons
- Nectarines
- Oranges
- Papayas
- Peaches
- Pears
- Pineapples
- Plums
- Persimmons

- Pomegranates
- Tangerines

Beverages

- Alcohol
- Caffeinated teas (except green tea)
- Coffee (caffeinated and decaffeinated)
- Energy drinks (including vitamin waters)
- Fruit juices
- Kefir
- Kombucha
- Sodas (diet or regular)
- Rice and soy milks

Condiments

Purchase condiments that are sugar and gluten-free and organic whenever possible. Condiments should be used sparingly and infrequently.

- Gravy
- Jams and jellies
- Ketchup
- Mayonnaise
- Mustard
- Pickles
- Relish
- Salad dressings
- Sauces with vinegars and sugar
- Soy sauce, pnzu and tamari sauce
- Spices that contain yeast, sugar or other additives

- Vinegars (except raw, unfiltered apple cider vinegar and unsweetened rice vinegar)
- Worcestershire sauce

Sweeteners

- Agave nectar
- Artificial sweeteners (aspartame, Nutrasweet, saccharin, acesulfame, and sucralose or Splenda)
- Barley malt
- Brown rice syrup
- Brown sugar
- Coconut sugar/nectar
- Corn syrup
- Dextrose Erythritol (Nectresse, Swerve, Truvia)
- Fructose (products sweetened with fruit juice)
- Honey (raw or processed)
- Maltitol
- Mannitol
- Maltodextrin
- Maple syrup
- Molasses
- Raw or evaporated cane juice
- Sorbitol
- White sugar
- Yacon syrup

Miscellaneous

- Cacao/chocolate (unless sweetened with stevia or xylitol)
- Candy
- Carob

- Cookies
- Donuts
- Fast food and fried foods
- Fermented foods (kimchi, sauerkraut, tempeh, yogurt, nutritional yeast, cultured vegetables)
- Fruit strips
- Gelatin
- Gum
- Jerky (beef or turkey)
- Lozenges/mints
- Muffins
- Pastries
- Pizza
- Processed food
- Smoked, dried, pickled, and cured foods

Pre-Conception Detoxification Instructions

Please note that these recommendations are only for pre-conception detoxification. Those who might be pregnant, are currently trying to conceive, or are breastfeeding should not follow a detoxification plan. Don't misunderstand—eating a clean, organic diet free of toxic, processed, and refined foods is good for everyone at any time. But only those who are not yet pregnant should be using fasting, juicing, or other detoxification methods to cleanse the body or specific systems within the body.

Detoxification is the process of clearing toxins from the body. An internal, natural elimination cycle occurs every night in each of us and continues through early morning. During this process, toxins are neutralized, modified, and eventually eliminated. For instance, the liver helps transform toxic substances while the blood carries waste products to the kidneys. The liver also moves wastes into the intestines where it is eliminated from the body via the stool. The proper elimination of these toxins and wastes is critical to maintaining good health and organ function. But when it becomes over-burdened by a diet high in toxins (sugar, gluten, chemicals, or processed or refined foods), oxidative stress, smoking, excessive alcohol use, and the like, we can assist the normal internal process by focusing our food intake on certain foods and eliminating others.

I also want to warn about excess detoxification. If you incorporate the food choices and other suggestions outlined below, it is not necessary to also do a fast, use laxatives, enemas, diuretics, or even excessive exercise. Too much detoxification can cause a loss of important nutrients such as protein or vitamin/mineral deficiencies.[3]

Below is a chart that will give you an idea of foods that cause congestion and foods that are detoxifying. Congestion-causing foods create congestion in the body's detoxification process. Focusing on supportive detoxification foods and eliminating congestion-causing foods for one to two weeks, can help clear mild congestion in the various internal systems that are responsible for detoxification.

Most Congesting versus Least Congesting

Most Congesting (Potentially More Toxic)						Least Congesting (More Detoxifying)
Fats		Sweets	Nuts	Rice	Roots	Fruits
Fried foods	Dairy	Organ meats	Seeds	Millet	Squashes	Greens
Hydrogenated fats		Refined flours	Oats	Vegetables		Water
Baked goods		Meats	Wheat	Potatoes		

(Haas & Levin, 2006 with modifications)

Adding any of the herbs, fruits, and vegetables below to a vegetable or protein smoothie each day for one to two weeks will give your drink an extra detoxification kick.

Cleanings Herbs

Burdock root. Skin and blood cleanser, diuretic, improves liver function, contains antibacterial and antifungal properties.

Cayenne pepper. Blood purifier.

Dandelion root. Liver and blood cleanser, diuretic, filters toxins.

Echinacea. Lymph cleanser, improves supports immune system.

Garlic. Blood cleanser, natural antibiotic.

Ginger root. Stimulates circulation and sweating.

Oregon grape root. Skin and colon cleanser, blood purifier, liver stimulant.

Parsley leaf. Diuretic, flushes kidneys.

Prickly ash bark. Good for nerves and joints, anti-infectious.

Sarsaparilla root. Blood and lymph cleanser, contains saponins, which reduce microbes and toxins.

Yellow dock root. Skin, blood, and liver cleanser contains vitamin C and iron.

(Haas & Levin, 2006)

Juices and Vegetables That Promote Detoxification

Apple. Liver, intestines.

Black cherry. Colon.

Grape. Colon.

Lemon. Liver, gallbladder.

Papaya. Stomach.

Beets. Blood, liver.

Pineapple. General inflammation and detoxification.

Celery. Kidneys.

Watermelon. Kidneys.

Beet greens.
Gallbladder, liver.

Cabbage. Colon.

Greens. Blood,
skin, intestines.

Potatoes. Intestines.

Spinach. Blood.

Garlic. Blood,
intestines, lymph.

Parsley. Kidneys.

Radish. Liver.

Watercress. Blood, skin.

Wheat grass. Liver,
intestines

(Haas, & Levin, 2006, with modifications)

Detoxifying Green Drink Recipe

For those of you dealing with a chronic health condition, poor bowel elimination, or other symptoms that indicate the need for more intense detoxification support, a more focused approach may be needed to get you cleaned out.

This green drink is packed full of detoxifying ingredients. Drink one to two 8-ounce servings per day for five to seven days, but start slow. On day one, drink 4 ounces and work up to the two servings per day gradually. If stomach or GI issues pop up, or if your bowel movements get too loose, cut back on the amount of green drink you are consuming or try eliminating the wheat grass during day one and two, adding it back in small quantities starting with day three. Each of us is biochemically different and will be impacted differently with a detoxification drink like this one.

Detoxifying Green Drink with Fruit Base

Use fresh, organic ingredients.

Prepare each serving fresh if possible to maximize nutrient value.

Start with 8 ounces of fresh pineapple or lemon juice in a high-powered blender that can liquefy vegetables.

Ingredients:

- 1 celery stalk with leaves
- Radish tops from 5 radishes
- Carrot top from 1 carrot
- ½ ounce burdock
- ½ ounce parsley
- ½ ounce chard

- ½ ounce plantain
- ½ ounce dandelion
- ½ ounce sprouts (pumpkin, bean, alfalfa)
- ½ ounce raspberry leaves
- ½ ounce wheatgrass

Blend until all ingredients are liquefied to suit your preferences and palate.

Optional: add ice to blender.

(Krohn & Taylor, 2000, with modifications)[4]

Antioxidant Salad Recipe

Free from Common Food Allergens

- Gluten
- Dairy
- Eggs
- Corn
- Soy
- Nightshades
- Nuts
- Sugar

Servings
Serves: 4 full salads
8 side salads

Ingredients

- 1 small head green cabbage
- 1 large red beet
- 1 bunch latticino kale
- ½ c pecan pieces
- ½ c robust olive oil
- ½ c kombucha (Recommended: GT Synergy Gingerberry)
- 1 lemon, juiced
- 1 tsp turmeric
- 1 tsp thyme
- 1 tsp. + more to taste Himalayan or Celtic sea salt
- ½ tsp. fine ground black pepper

Directions

1. Using a hand grater or food processor, shred the cabbage and grate the beet. Remove the ribs from the kale and coarsely chop into bite-size pieces.
2. In a large mixing bowl, combine the cabbage, beets, kale, and pecans.
3. In a small mixing bowl, whisk together the olive oil, kombucha, lemon juice, turmeric, thyme, salt, and pepper. Drizzle the dressing over the cabbage mix and toss to evenly coat.
4. Chill and serve as a cold, raw salad.

Notes

Option to serve as a warm salad by placing salad in a large sauté pan and cook for 5–8 minutes, or until vegetables are al dente.

Contributed by Rebekah Fedrowitz, MDN, BCHN
www.youarewellhealth.com
© 2017 You *AreWell^TM*
Used with permission.[5]

List of Cruciferous Vegetables

Due to the goitrogenic properties that can affect the thyroid gland, cruciferous vegetables should be lightly steamed or cooked.

- Arugula
- Bok choy
- Broccoli
- Brussels sprouts
- Cabbage
- Cauliflower
- Chinese cabbage
- Collard greens
- Daikon radish
- Horseradish
- Kale
- Kohlrabi
- Land cress
- Mustard greens
- Radish
- Rutabaga
- Shepherd's purse
- Turnip
- Watercress

(Mateljan, 2007)[6]

Sources of Gluten

Gluten-Containing Grains and Their Derivatives

- Wheat
- Varieties and derivatives of wheat such as:
  - wheatberries
  - durum
  - emmer
  - semolina
  - spelt
  - farina
  - farro
  - graham
  - KAMUT® khorasan wheat
  - einkorn wheat
- Rye
- Barley
- Triticale
- Malt in various forms including malted barley flour, malted milk or milkshakes, malt extract, malt syrup, malt flavoring, and malt vinegar.
- Brewer's Yeast
- Wheat Starch that has not been processed to remove the presence of gluten to below 20 parts per million (ppm) and adhere to the FDA Labeling Law.*

*According to the FDA, if a food contains wheat starch, it may only be labeled gluten-free if that product has been processed to remove gluten and tests below 20 ppm of gluten. With the enactment of this law on August 5th, 2014, individuals with celiac disease or gluten intolerance can be assured that a food containing wheat starch and labeled gluten-free contains no more than 20 ppm of gluten. If a product labeled gluten-free contains wheat starch in the ingredient list, it must be followed by an asterisk explaining that the wheat has been processed sufficiently to adhere to the FDA requirements for gluten-free labeling.

Common Foods That Contain Gluten

- Pastas
  - ravioli, dumplings, couscous, and gnocchi
- Noodles
  - ramen, udon, soba (those made with only a percentage of buckwheat flour) chow mein, and egg noodles. (Note: Rice noodles and mung bean noodles are gluten-free.)
- Breads and Pastries
  - croissants, pita, naan, bagels, flatbreads, cornbread, potato bread, muffins, donuts, rolls.
- Crackers
  - pretzels, Goldfish, graham crackers
- Baked Goods
  - cakes, cookies, pie crusts, brownies
- Cereal & Granola
  - corn flakes and rice puffs often contain malt extract/flavoring, and granola is often made with regular oats, not gluten-free oats
- Breakfast Foods
  - pancakes, waffles, French toast, crepes, and biscuits
- Breading & Coating Mixes
  - panko breadcrumbs
- Croutons
  - stuffings, dressings

- Sauces & Gravies (many use wheat flour as a thickener)
  - traditional soy sauce, cream sauces made with a roux
- Flour tortillas
- Beer (unless explicitly gluten-free) and any malt beverages (see "Distilled Beverages and Vinegars" below for more information on alcoholic beverages)
- Brewer's Yeast
  - Anything else that uses "wheat flour" as an ingredient

Foods That May Contain Gluten (verified by reading the label or checking with the manufacturer or provider)

- Energy bars/granola bars—some bars may contain wheat as an ingredient, and most use oats that are not gluten-free.
- French fries—be careful of batter containing wheat flour or cross-contact from fryers.
- Potato chips—some potato chip seasonings may contain malt vinegar or wheat starch.
- Processed lunch meats
- Candy and candy bars
- Soup—pay special attention to cream-based soups, which have flour as a thickener. Many soups also contain barley.
- Multi-grain or "artisan" tortilla chips or tortillas that are not entirely corn-based may contain a wheat-based ingredient.
- Salad dressings and marinades—may contain malt vinegar, soy sauce, flour.
- Starch or dextrin if found on a meat or poultry product could be from any grain, including wheat.

- Brown rice syrup—may be made with barley enzymes.
- Meat substitutes made with seitan (wheat gluten) such as vegetarian burgers, vegetarian sausage, imitation bacon, imitation seafood. (Note: Tofu is gluten-free, but be cautious of soy sauce marinades and cross-contact when eating out, especially when the tofu is fried.)
- Soy sauce (Though tamari made without wheat is gluten-free.)
- Self-basting poultry
- Pre-seasoned meats
- Cheesecake filling—some recipes include wheat flour.
- Eggs served at restaurants—some restaurants put pancake batter in their scrambled eggs and omelets, but on their own, eggs are naturally gluten-free.

Distilled Beverages and Vinegars

Most *distilled* alcoholic beverages and vinegars are gluten-free. These distilled products do not contain any harmful gluten peptides even if they are made from gluten-containing grains. Research indicates that the gluten peptide is too large to carry over in the distillation process, leaving the resulting liquid gluten-free.

Wines and hard liquor/distilled beverages are gluten-free. However, *beers, ales, lagers, malt beverages, and malt vinegars that are made from gluten-containing grains are not distilled and therefore are not gluten-free.* There are several brands of gluten-free beers available in the United States and abroad.

Other Items That Must Be Verified by Reading the Label or Checking with the Manufacturer

- **Lipstick**, **lip-gloss**, and **lip balm** because they are unintentionally ingested
- **Communion wafers**
- **Herbal or nutritional supplements**
- **Drugs and over-the-counter medications**
- **Vitamins and supplements**
- **Play-Doh**: Children may touch their mouths or eat after handling wheat-based Play-Doh. For a safer alternative, make a homemade version with gluten-free flour.

Label-Reading

Products labeled wheat-free are not necessarily gluten-free. They may still contain spelt (a form of wheat), rye, or barley-based ingredients that are not gluten-free. To confirm if something is gluten-free, be sure to refer to the product's ingredient list.

Cross-Contact

When preparing gluten-free foods, it is important to avoid cross-contact. Cross-contact occurs when foods or ingredients come into contact with gluten, generally through shared utensils or a shared cooking/storage environment. In order for food to be safe for someone with celiac disease, it must not come into contact with food containing gluten.

Places where cross-contact can occur:

- Toasters used for both gluten-free and regular bread.
- Colanders
- Cutting boards
- Flour sifters
- Deep fried foods cooked in oil shared with breaded products.
- Shared containers including improperly washed containers.
- Condiments such as butter, peanut butter, jam, mustard, and mayonnaise may become contaminated when utensils used on gluten-containing food are double-dipped.
- Wheat flour can stay airborne for many hours in a bakery (or at home) and contaminate exposed preparation surfaces and utensils or uncovered gluten-free products.
- Oats—cross-contact can occur in the field when oats are grown side-by-side with wheat; select only oats specifically labeled gluten-free.
- Pizza—pizzerias that offer gluten-free crusts sometimes do not control for cross-contact with their wheat-based doughs.
- French fries
- Non-certified baked goods, e.g., "gluten-free" goods from otherwise gluten-containing bakeries.
- Bulk bins at grocery stores or co-ops.

Source: Celiac Disease Foundation® (2017). Retrieved 10-29-17 from https://celiac.org/live-gluten-free/glutenfreediet/sources-of-gluten/

Summary of Daily Recommended Food Servings

<u>Dairy</u>
Daily and weekly recommendations:

- Dairy products are part of the protein food group.
- Dairy should be consumed in small quantities or eliminated.
- If choosing dairy products, always purchase organic, antibiotic-free and hormone-free, and from grass-fed livestock.
- For cow-milk substitutes, consider unsweetened hemp, almond, or coconut milks.

<u>Omega-3 and -6 Fats</u>
Daily and weekly recommendations:

- Consume 340 grams (two 6-ounce servings) per week of seafood. or high-quality, grass-fed beef. (See food lists in Chapter 4.)
- Focus on a combination of omega-3 food sources and a high-quality fish-oil supplement to ensure you reach the proper amount of DHA fats, approximately 600 mg or more per day.
- Important to limit seafood intake to wild-caught only to avoid exposure to mercury toxicity or other neuro-toxins. Avoid types of fish known to be high in mercury and other toxins (shellfish, shark, swordfish, king mackerel, tilefish, marlin, orange roughy, and tuna).
- Consume high-quality, organic, grass-fed beef or bison up to three times per week.

- Include a high-quality EPA/DHA fish-oil supplement with your supplement regiment.
- Avoid using fats and oils with high omega-6 content. (See food lists in Chapter 4.)
- Include a high-quality EPA/DHA fish-oil supplement with your supplement regiment, minimum of 600 mg per day of DHA.
- Avoid using fats and oils with high omega-6 content. (See food list).

Proteins
Daily Recommendations:

- Protein should make up approximately 25 percent of daily diet, 60–75 grams of protein per day during first trimester.
- Protein sources should be varied and include organic eggs and high-quality, organic meats and fish (wild-caught).

Grains
Daily recommendations:

- Gluten-free grains should make up less than 1 percent of daily diet, or one small serving per day (examples: one slice of gluten-free bread, four or five crackers, one-half cup of gluten-free pasta).
- Choose products that are made with gluten-free grains.
- If blood sugar issues are present or other health concerns, limit gluten-free grains to maximum of three times per week.

Vegetables
Daily recommendations:

- Starchy vegetables should make up no more than two servings per day of total vegetable intake, or no more than 5 percent of daily diet. If blood sugar issues are present, starchy vegetables should be reduced to three or four times per week.
- A vegetable is considered high in starch if it contains more than 5 grams of carbohydrates per half-cup.
- Choose vegetables from organic sources
- Consume legumes only after soaking and cooking

Daily recommendations:

- Non-starchy vegetables should make up 60 percent of daily diet.
- Choose vegetables from organic sources
- Eat a variety of vegetables.
- Consume at least 5 servings or 2 ½ cups of non-starchy vegetables per day, a minimum of one with each meal.
- A portion of daily vegetable intake can be liquefied in a high-powered blender and consumed by drinking. See vegetable juice recipe in this section.
- Eat vegetables barely cooked (crunchy texture) as often as possible, except for spinach, Swiss chard and beet greens, which should be thoroughly steamed or boiled to minimize the oxalate content (Mateljan, 2007).

Fruits

Daily recommendations:

- Fruits should make up no more than 10 percent of daily diet.
- One or two servings per day of low-glycemic fruits
- One serving per day of moderate-glycemic fruit
- High-glycemic fruits should be consumed in small quantities (¼ cup) and only on an occasional basis as a snack or dessert.

ENDNOTES

Introduction

[1]   "U.S. Fertility Rates Hit Record Low in 2013…and 2006…and 1976," *PEW Research Center*, last modified February 24, 2015, http://www.pewresearch.org/fact-tank/2018/01/18/is-u-s-fertility-at-an-all-time-low-it-depends/ft_15-02-18_fertility-2/.

[2]   "Who Gets MS?" *National Multiple Sclerosis Society*, 2016, accessed March 10, 2016, https://www.nationalmssociety.org/What-is-MS/Who-Gets-MS.

[3]   Ann Boroch, *The Candida Cure*. (Quintessential Healing Publishing, Inc, 2015.)

[4]   "Frequently Asked Questions." *MSAA: The Multiple Sclerosis Association of America*, accessed April 10, 2017, https://mymsaa.org/ms-information/faqs/.

[5]   "U.S. Fertility Rates."

[6]   Marco Noventa et al., "May Underdiagnosed Nutrition Imbalances Be Responsible for a Portion of So-Called Unexplained Infertility? From Diagnosis to Potential Treatment Options." *Reproductive Sciences* 23, no. 6 (2015): 812–822, accessed April 2017, doi:10.1177/1933719115620496.

[7]   John J. Bromfield et al., "Maternal Tract Factors Contribute to Paternal Seminal Fluid Impact on Metabolic Phenotype

in Offspring," *Proceedings of the National Academy of Sciences*, February 11, 2014, http://www.pnas.org/content/111/6/2200.

Chapter 1

1   Justin Caba, "Seminal Fluid, Not Just Sperm, Plays a Role in the Fetus' Health, Including Obesity and Diabetes," *Medical Daily*, January 28, 2014, accessed April 5, 2017, http://www.medicaldaily.com/seminal-fluid-not-just-sperm-plays-role-fetus-health-including-obesity-and-diabetes-268040.

2   Bromfield et al., "Maternal Tract."

3   "U.S. Fertility Rates."

4   "U.S. Fertility Rates."

5   "U.S. Fertility Rates..."; M. Nathaniel Mead, "Nutrigenomics: The Genome–Food Interface," *Environmental Health Perspectives* 115, no. 12 (2007), doi:10.1289/ehp.115-a582.

6   Mead, "Nutrigenomics."

7   Stephen Guyenet, "Fat, Added Fat, and Obesity in America," *Whole Health Source: Nutrition and Health Science* (web log), November 22, 2015, accessed April 4, 2017, http://wholehealthsource.blogspot.com/2015/11/fat-added-fat-and-obesity-in-america.html.

8   Iva Keene, "10 Ways to Address Your Root Causes of Infertility Naturally," *Mercola.com*, October 14, 2009, accessed June 13, 2015, https://blogs.mercola.com/sites/vitalvotes/archive/2009/10/14/10-Ways-to-Address-Your-Root-Causes-of-Infertility--Naturally.aspx.

9   Kris Gunnars, "11 Graphs That Show Everything That Is Wrong With the Modern Diet," *Healthline*, June 8, 2017. https://www.healthline.com/nutrition/11-graphs-that-show-what-is-wrong-with-modern-diet.

10   Gunnars, "11 Graphs."

11   Henry Blodget, "American Per-Capita Sugar Consumption Hits 100 Pounds Per Year," *Business Insider*, February 19, 2012, accessed April 4, 2017, http://www.businessinsider.com/chart-american-sugar-consumption-2012-2.

12   Gunnars, "11 Graphs."

13   Gunnars, "11 Graphs."

14   Gunnars, "11 Graphs."

15   Gunnars, "11 Graphs."

16   Alexander Gaffney, "How Many Drugs Has FDA Approved in its Entire History? New Paper Explains," *Regulatory Affairs Professionals Society*, October 3, 2014, https://www.raps.org/regulatory-focus%E2%84%A2/news-articles/2014/10/how-many-drugs-has-fda-approved-in-its-entire-history-new-paper-explains.

17   Gunnars, "11 Graphs."

18   Gunnars, "11 Graphs."

19   "Significant Dates in U.S. Food and Drug Law History," *U.S. Food and Drug Administration*, 2015, accessed July 2, 2015, http://www.fda.gov/aboutFDA/whatwedo/history/milestones/ucm128305.htm.

20   Keene, "10 Ways."

21   American Nutrition Association, review of *Excitotoxins: The Taste That Kills*, by R. Blaylock, Nutrition Digest 38, no. 1 (2015).

22   Autoimmunity Research Foundation, "Incidence and Prevalence of Chronic Disease," *The Marshall Protocol Knowledge Base*, 2015, accessed April 4, 2017, https://mpkb.org/home/pathogenesis/epidemiology.

23   R. Mason, "Optimal Therapeutic Strategy for Treating Patients with Hypertension and Athlerosclerosis: Focus on Olmesartan Medoxomil," *National Institutes of Health*, 2011, doi:10.2147/VHRM.S20737; "Alternative Medicine Taking Hold among Americans: Report," *HealthDay News*, 2016, accessed April 10, 2017, https://consumer.healthday.com.

24   Nahin and Stephanie Romanoff, *National Health Statistics Reports*, June 22, 2016.

25   J. Bland, *The Institute for Functional Medicine*, 2016, https://www.ifm.org.

Chapter 2

1   Judith R. Brower, "A Crash Course in Epigenetics Part 1: An Intro to Epigenetics," *Bitesize Bio*, January 16, 2017, accessed April 11, 2017, https://bitesizebio.com/8807/.

2   National Center for Health Statistics, Center for Disease Control and Prevention, updated February 2015.

3   National Center for Health Statistics.

4   Naina Kumar and Amit Kant Singh, "Trends of Male Factor Infertility, an Important Cause of Infertility: A Review of Literature," *Journal of Reproductive Sciences* 8, no. 4 (2015): 191–196, accessed May 22, 2016, http://www.jhrsonline. org/article.asp?issn=0974-1208;year=2015;volume=8;issue=4;spage=191;epage=196;aulast=Kumar.

5   Victor M. Brugh III and Larry I. Lipschultz, "Male Factor Infertility," *Medical Clinics* 88, no. 2 (2004): 367–385, accessed April 12, 2017, www.medical.theclinics.com/article/S0025-7125(03)00150-0/fulltext.

6   G. Gnoth et al., "Time to Pregnancy: Results of the German Prospective Study and Impact on the Management of Infertility," *Human Reproduction* 18, no. 9 (September 2003): 1959–1966, doi.org/10.1093/humrep/deg366.

7   National Institute of Environmental Health Sciences, "Don't Turn to Assisted Reproduction Too Quickly Warns US Expert," 2002, accessed June 17, 2016 https://www.niehs.nih.gov/news/newsroom/releases/2002/july03/index.cfm

8   Michael Murray and Joseph Pizzorno, *The Encyclopedia of Natural Medicine* (London: Simon & Schuster, 2014).

9   Murray and Pizzorno, *Encyclopedia.*

10 "Endometriosis," *American Congress of Gynecologists,* 2014, accessed June 17, 2016, https://www.acog.org/-/media/For%20Patients/faq013.pdf?dmc=1&ts=20140605T1007118112.

11 "Dysmenorrhea," *American Congress of Gynecologists,* 2014, accessed June, 17, 2016, https://www.acog.org/-/media/For-Patients/faq046.pdf?dmc=1&ts=20180227T1758530193.

12 H. Teede, A. Deeks, and L. Moran, BMC Medicine, 2010, accessed June 17, 2018, "Polycystic ovary syndrome: a complex condition with psychological, reproductive and metabolic manifestations that impacts on health across the lifespan" https://bmcmedicine.biomedcentral.com/articles/10.1186/1741-7015-8-1.

13 Murray and Pizzorno, *Encyclopedia.*

14 Murray and Pizzorno, *Encyclopedia.*

15 Brugh and Lipschultz, "Male Factor Infertility."

16 Richard M. Sharpe, "Environmental/Lifestyle Effects on Spermatogenesis," *Philosophical Transactions of the Royal Society B* 365, no. 1546 (2010) 1697–1712, accessed June 17, 2016, doi: 10.1098/rstb.2009.0206, http://rstb.royalsocietypublishing.org/content/365/1546/1697.short.

17 Murray and Pizzorno, *Encyclopedia.*

18 Murray and Pizzorno, *Encyclopedia.*

19 Murray and Pizzorno, *Encyclopedia.*

20 "The Best Fertility Apps of 2017," *Healthline Media,* 2016, accessed October 3, 2017, www.healthline.com/health/pregnancy/fertility-apps#Intro1.

Chapter 3

1 M. Gershon, *The Second Brain* (New York: HarperCollins Publishers, 1998/2013).

2 "Human Microbiome: The Role of Microbes in Human Health," *American Museum of Natural History,* 2016, accessed June 12, 2017, https://www.amnh.org/content/download/131242/2201977/file/human_microbiome_the_role_of_microbes_in_human_health_stepread1.pdf

3   *American Museum of Natural History* (2016). "Human Microbiome."

4   T. Harmon and A. Wakeford, *Your Baby's Microbiome* (White River Junction, Vermont: Chelsea Green Publishing, 2017).

5   Harmon and Wakeford, *Your Baby's Microbiome.*

6   Harmon and Wakeford, *Your Baby's Microbiome.*

7   Jane A. Foster, "Gut Feelings: Bacteria and the Brain," NIH. *Cerebrum. The Dana Forum on Brain Science* 2013, no. 9 (July–August 2013), accessed June 12, 2017, https://www.ncbi.nlm.nih.gov/pmc/articles/PMC3788166/.

8   "NIH Human Microbiome Project Defines Normal Bacterial Makeup of the Body," *National Institutes of Health*, 2012, accessed June 9, 2016, http://www.nih.gov/news/health/jun2012/nhgri-13.htm.

9   Keesha Ewers, *Solving the Autoimmune Puzzle: The Woman's Guide to Reclaiming Emotional Freedom and Vibrant Health* (Issaquah, WA: Samadhi Press, 2017).

10   R. Bowers et al., "Sources of Bacteria in Outdoor Air Across Cities in the Midwestern United States," *Applied and Environmental Microbiology* 77, no. 18 (2011).

11   Foster, "Gut Feelings."

12   Foster, "Gut Feelings."

13   G. Clarke et al., "Priming for Health: Gut Microbiota Acquired in Early Life Regulates Physiology, Brain and Behaviour," *Acta Paediatr* 103 (2014): 812–819, doi:10.1111/apa.12674.

14   "NIH Human Microbiome."

15   "NIH Human Microbiome"; NIH, *The Human Microbiome, Diet, and Health: Workshop Summary* (Washington, D.C.: National Academies Press [US], 2013).

16   A. Srinivasan, J. Lopez-Ribot, and A. Ramasubramanian, "Microscale Microbial Culture," *Future Microbiology* 10, no. 2 (2015), doi 10.2217/fmb.14.129; "NIH Human Microbiome."

17   K. Krautkramer and F. Rey, "Gut's Microbial Community Shown to Influence Host Gene Expression," *University of Wisconsin-Madison, School and Medicine and Public Health*, accessed June 10, 2017, http://www.med.wisc.edu/news-events/guts-microbial-community-shown-to-influence-host-gene-expression/49718.

18   "NIH Human Microbiome."

19   Krautkramer,   Lopez-Ribot,   and   Ramasubramanian, "Microscale."

20   "NIH Human Microbiome."

21   Joseph Mercola, "Research Reveals the Importance of Your Microbiome for Optimal Health," *Mercola,* July 13, 2013, accessed June 10, 2017, http://articles.mercola.com/sites/articles/archive/2015/07/13/importance-gut-microbiome.aspx.

22   *Mercola,* "Research Reveals."

23   *Mercola,* "Research Reveals."

24   D. Perlmutter, *Brain Maker* (New York: Little, Brown and Company, 2015).

25   Mercola, "Research Reveals."

26   A. G. Braundemeier et al., "Individualized Medicine and the Microbiome in Reproductive Tract," *Frontiers in Physiology* 6, no. 97 (2015), http://doi.org/10.3389/fphys.2015.00097.

27   Braundemeier et al., "Individualized Medicine."

28   Braundemeier et al., "Individualized Medicine."

29   T. Shin and H. Okada, "Infertility in Men with Inflammatory Bowel Disease," *World Journal of Gastrointestinal Pharmacology and Therapeutics* 7, no. 3 (2016): 361–369, http://doi.org/10.4292/wjgpt.v7.i3.361.

30   Jason M. Franasiak, M.D. and Richard T. Scott, Jr., M.D., "Microbiome in Human Reproduction," *American Society for Reproductive Medicine, Fertility and Sterility Journal* 104, no. 6. (December 2015): 0015–0282, accessed June 10, 2017, http://www.fertstert.org/article/S0015-0282(15)02032-4/abstract.

31   Harmon and Wakeford, *Your Baby's Microbiome.*

32   A. Park, "Babies in the Womb Aren't So Sterile After All," *TIME*, December 28, 2015, http://time.com/4159249/baby-microbiome-womb/.

33   Park, "Babies."

34   Harmon and Wakeford, *Your Baby's Microbiome.*

35   Harmon and Wakeford, *Your Baby's Microbiome.*

36   N. T. Mueller et al., "The Infant Microbiome Development: Mom Matters," *Trends in Molecular Medicine* 21, no. 2 (2014): 109–117, http://doi.org/10.1016/j.molmed.2014.12.002; S. J. Song, M. G. Dominguez-Bello, and R. Knight, "How Delivery Mode and Feeding Can Shape the Bacterial Community in the Infant Gut," CMAJ Canadian Medical Association Journal 185, no. 5 (2013): 373–374, http://doi.org/10.1503/cmaj.130147; "The Amazing Benefits of Breastfeeding," *Mercola*, accessed June 2, 2017, http://articles.mercola.com/sites/articles/archive/2016/01/02/amazsing-benefits-breastfeeding.aspx.

37   Harmon and Wakeford, *Your Baby's Microbiome.*

38   Harmon and Wakeford, *Your Baby's Microbiome.*

39   Song, Dominguez-Bello, and Knight, "How Delivery Mode."

40   Song, Dominguez-Bello, and Knight, "How Delivery Mode."

41   Harmon and Wakeford, *Your Baby's Microbiome.*

Chapter 4

1   K. McGuire and K. Beerman, *Nutritional Sciences, Third Edition* (Belmont, California: Cengage Learning, 2013).

2   McGuire and Beerman, *Nutritional Sciences.*

3   McGuire and Beerman, *Nutritional Sciences.*

4   McGuire and Beerman, *Nutritional Sciences.*

5   K. M. Rasmussen and A. L. Yaktine, eds., *Weight Gain during Pregnancy: Reexaming the Guidelines* (Washington, D.C.: National Academies Press [US], 2009).

6   G. Mateljan, *The World's Healthiest Foods* (Seattle: WHFoods, 2007).

7   G. Smith "Nightshades," *The Weston A. Price Foundation*, March 20, 2010, accessed June 9, 2016, www.westonaprice. org/health-topics/nightshades/.

8   Smith, "Nightshades."

9   McGuire and Beerman, *Nutritional Sciences.*

10   McGuire and Beerman, *Nutritional Sciences.*

11   McGuire and Beerman, *Nutritional Sciences*; Rasmussen and Yaktine, *Weight Gain.*

12   Rasmussen and Yaktine, *Weight Gain.*

13   Rasmussen and Yaktine, *Weight Gain.*

14   Rasmussen and Yaktine, *Weight Gain.*

15   Rasmussen and Yaktine, *Weight Gain.*

16   Rasmussen and Yaktine, *Weight Gain.*

17   E. Fawcett, J. Fawcett, and D. Mamanian, "A Meta-Analysis of the Worldwide Prevalence of Pica during Pregnancy and the Postpartum Period," *International Journal of Gynecology. & Obstetrics.*, June 2016, accessed June 19, 2016, PMID: 26892693, https://www.ncbi.nlm.nih.gov/pubmed/26892693.

18   Fawcett, Fawcett, and Mazmanian, "A Meta-Analysis."

19   Fawcett, Fawcett, and Mazmanian, "A Meta-Analysis."

20   Murray, *The Encyclopedia of Healing Foods* (New York: Atria Books, 2005).

21   Murray, *The Encyclopedia of Healing Foods.*

22   "Gestational Diabetes—Diabetes during Pregnancy," *Endocrineweb*, updated April 2016, accessed June 9, 2016, www.endocrineweb. com/conditions/gestation-diabetes/gestation-diabetes.

23   P. Soma-Pillay et al., "Physiological Changes in Pregnancy," *Cardiovascular Journal of Africa* 27, no. 2 (2016): 89–94, http:// doi.org/10.5830/CVJA-2016-021.

24   Soma-Pillay et al., "Physiological Changes."

25   Soma-Pillay et al., "Physiological Changes."

26   "Gestational Diabetes."

27   "Gestational Diabetes."

28   "Gestational Diabetes."

29   "Gestational Diabetes."

30   "What Is the Glycemic Index?" *Glycemic-Index.org*, 2016, accessed June 14, 2016, glycemic-index.org.

31   "What Is the Glycemic Index?"

32   "What Is the Glycemic Index?"

33   G. Mateljan, *The World's Healthiest Foods* (Seattle: WHFoods, 2007).

34   G. Mateljan, *The World's Healthiest Foods* (Seattle: WHFoods, 2007).

35   Amy Myers, "The Dangers of Dairy," *Mind Body Green*, accessed February 10, 2017, https://www.mindbodygreen.com/0-8646/the-dangers-of-dairy.html.

36   Myers, "The Dangers."

37   Myers, "The Dangers."

38   McGuire and Beerman, *Nutritional Sciences*.

39   Jaclyn M. Coletta, M.D., Stacey J. Bell, DSc, RD, and Ashley S. Roman, M.D., "Omega-3 Fatty Acids and Pregnancy," NIH, *Journal of Obstetrics & Gynecology* 3, no. 4 (2010), accessed June 9, 2016, https://www.ncbi.nlm.nih.gov/pmc/articles/PMC3046737.

40   Jaclyn M. Coletta, M.D., Stacey J. Bell, DSc, RD, and Ashley S. Roman, M.D., "Omega-3 Fatty Acids and Pregnancy," NIH, *Journal of Obstetrics & Gynecology* 3, no. 4 (2010), accessed June 9, 2016, https://www.ncbi.nlm.nih.gov/pmc/articles/PMC3046737.

41   Coletta, Bell, and Roman, "Omega-3."

42   T. Wahls, *The Wahls Protocol* (New York: Penguin Group Random House, 2014).

43   Coletta, Bell, and Roman, "Omega-3."

44   Coletta, Bell, and Roman, "Omega-3."

45   Wahls, *The Wahls Protocol*.

46   Coletta, Bell, and Roman, "Omega-3."; James A. Greenberg, M.D., Stacey J. Bell, DSc, RD, and Wendy Van Ausdal. "Omega-3 Fatty Acid Supplementation during Pregnancy," *Journal of Obstetrics & Gynecology* 1, no. 4 (Fall 2008):

162–169, https://www.ncbi.nlm.nih.gov/pmc/articles/PMC2621042/#!po=29.2857.

47 Coletta, Bell, and Roman, "Omega-3."

48 Coletta, Bell, and Roman, "Omega-3."

49 D. Schwarzbein, The Schwarzbein Principle II (Deerfield Beach: Health Communications Inc., 2002).

50 Coletta, Bell, and Roman, "Omega-3."

51 McGuire and Beerman, *Nutritional Sciences*.

52 Coletta, Bell, and Roman, "Omega-3."

53 G. Mateljan, *The World's Healthiest Foods* (Seattle: WHFoods, 2007).

54 EPA-FDA, "2017 EPA-FDA Advice about Eating Fish and Shellfish," accessed February 10, 2017. https://www.epa.gov/fish-tech/2017-epa-fda-advice-about-eating-fish-and-shellfish.

55 G. Mateljan, *The World's Healthiest Foods* (Seattle: WHFoods, 2007).

56 G. Mateljan, *The World's Healthiest Foods* (Seattle: WHFoods, 2007).

57 A. Carroccio et al. "Non-Celiac Wheat Sensitivity Diagnosed by Double-Blind Placebo-Controlled Challenge"; G. Mateljan, *The World's Healthiest Foods* (Seattle: WHFoods, 2007); Exploring a New Clinical Entity," *Am J Gastroenterol* 107, no. 12 (2012): 1898–906; R. M. Beery Marchiono and J. W. Birk, "Wheat-Related Disorders Reviewed: Making a Grain of Sense," *Gastroenterol Hepatol* (2014).

58 Perlmutter, *Grain Brain* (New York: Little, Brown and Company, 2013).

59 "Celiac Disease and Non-Celiac Gluten Sensitivity," *LifeExtension.com*, 2017, accessed October 26, 2017, www.lifeextension.com/protocols/gastrointestinal/celiac-disease-and-non-celiac-gluten-sensitivity/page-02.

60 Perlmutter, *Grain Brain*.

61 Perlmutter, *Grain Brain*.

62 Perlmutter, *Grain Brain*.

63   "Celiac Disease and Non-Celiac Gluten Sensitivity," LifeExtension.com, 2017, accessed October 26, 2017, www.lifeextension.com/protocols/gastrointestinal/celiac-disease-and-non-celiac-gluten-sensitivity/page-02.

64   G. Mateljan, *The World's Healthiest Foods* (Seattle: WHFoods, 2007).

65   Murray, *The Encyclopedia of Healing Foods.*

66   Murray, *The Encyclopedia of Healing Foods.*

67   Murray, *The Encyclopedia of Healing Foods.*

68   G. Mateljan, *The World's Healthiest Foods* (Seattle: WHFoods, 2007).

69   G. Mateljan, *The World's Healthiest Foods* (Seattle: WHFoods, 2007).

70   L. Turner, "Find Hormonal Harmony & Counteract Xenoestrogens Naturally," *Better Nutrition*, accessed June 13, 2015, www.betternutrition.com/xenoestrogensenvironmentalhormones/.

71   Mateljan, *The World's.*

72   Mateljan, *The World's.*

73   Schwarzbein, *The Schwarzbein.*

74   Mateljan, *The World's.*

75   "What's in Your Condiments?" *Mercola,* 2013, accessed March 4, 2017. https://articles.mercola.com/sites/articles/archive/2013/08/12/condiments.aspx.

76   Coletta, Bell, and Roman, "Omega-3."

77   Coletta, Bell, and Roman, "Omega-3."

78   EPA-FDA, "2017."

79   EPA-FDA, "2017."

80   Mateljan, *The World's.*

Chapter 5

1   "The Importance of Folate, Zin and Antioxidants in the Pathogenesis and Prevention of Subfertility," *Oxford Journals, Human Reproduction Update* 13, no. 2 (March/April 2007):

163–172, accessed May 23, 2016, https://humupd.oxfordjournals.org/content/13/2/163.short.

2   T. Scott, *The Antianxiety Food Solution* (Oakland: New Harbinger Publications, Inc., 2011).

3   "Fluoride and Other Chemicals in Your Drinking Water Could Be Wrecking Your Health," *Mercola*, 2013, accessed May 23, 2016, https://articles.mercola.com/sites/articles/archive/2013/12/28/fluoride-drinking-water.aspx.

4   *Mercola*, "Fluoride."

5   "Toxins in Our Drinking Water," *Global Healing Center,* 2016, accessed May 23, 2016, www.globalhealingcenter.com/water/water-toxins.

6   E. H, Ruder et al., "Oxidative Stress and Antioxidants: Exposure and Impact on Female Fertility," *NIH, Human Reproduction Update* 14, no. 4 (July–August 2008): 345–357.

7   "The Importance of Folate."

8   A. Agarwal, S. Gupta, and R. Sharma, "Role of Oxidative Stress in Female Reproduction," *Reproductive Biology and Endocrinology* (July 2005).

9   "Vitamin D Has Been Shown to Dramatically Improve Fertility," *Mercola*, 2012, accessed May 24, 2016, https://articles.mercola.com/sites/articles/archive/2012/02/16/the-vitamin-that-has-been-shown-to-dramatically-improve-infertility.aspx.

10   J. E. Chavarro et al., "Iron Intake and Risk of Ovulatory Infertility," NIH, Obstetrics Gynecology 108, no. 5 (2006): 1145–1152.

11   C. Woodham, "Trouble Trying to Conceive? This May Be Why," *Massachusetts General Hospital*, 2012, accessed May 23, 2016, https://health.usnews.com/health-news/articles/2012/06/06/trouble-trying-to-conceive-this-may-be-why.

12   Woodham, "Trouble."

13   M. Bastuba, "How Caffeine, Alcohol and Tobacco Affect Male Fertility," (web log) 2011, accessed

March 16, 2017, https://www.malefertility.md/blog/how-caffeine-alcohol-and-tobacco-affect-male-fertility.

14 "Men with High Levels of This Have 4 Times Lower Sperm Count," *Mercola*, 2011, accessed May 23, 2016, www.mercola.com/sites/articles/archieve/2011/03/08/7-surprising-sperm-killers-that-could-leave-men-shooting-blanks.aspx.

15 *Mercola*, "Men with."

16 "Stress Degrades Sperm Quality, Study Shows," *Journal of Fertility and Sterility*, (2014), accessed May 23, 2016. www.ASRM.org/fertilityandsterility/.

17 *Mercola*, "Vitamin D."

18 *Mercola*, "Vitamin D."

19 B. H. Malecki, B. Tartibian, and Chehrazi, "The Effects of Three Different Exercise Modalities on Markers of Male Reproduction in Healthy Subjects: A Randomized Controlled Trial," *Society for Reproduction and Fertility*, (2016), doi: 10.1530/REP-16-0318.

20 Maleki, Tartibian, and Chehrazi, "The Effects."

21 Maleki, Tartibian, and Chehrazi, "The Effects."

22 Maleki, Tartibian, and Chehrazi, "The Effects."

23 Agarwal, Ashok et al. "Effects of radiofrequency electromagnetic waves (RF-EMW) from cellular phones on human ejaculated semen: an in vitro pilot study" *Fertility and Sterility* (2009), doi:10.1016/j.fertnstert.2008.08.022.

24 Coletta, Bell, and Roman, "Omega-3."

25 Coletta, Bell, and Roman, "Omega-3."

26 EPA-FDA, "2017."

27 Mateljan, *The World's*.

28 E. Haas and B. Levin, *Staying Healthy with Nutrition* (New York: Random House, 2006), 576.

Chapter 6

1 A. J. Romm, *The Natural Pregnancy Book* (New York: Ten Speed Press, division of Random House, rev. 2014).

2 Cleveland Clinic, "Fetal Development: Stages of Growth," 2016, accessed March 4, 2017, https://my.clevelandclinic.org/health/articles/fetal-development-stages-of-growth.

3 Cleveland Clinic, "Fetal Development."

4 Cleveland Clinic, "Fetal Development."

5 Cleveland Clinic, "Fetal Development."

6 Cleveland Clinic, "Fetal Development."

7 Romm, *The Natural.*

8 U.S. Department of Health and Human Services, "Stages of Pregnancy," 2017, accessed March 4, 2017. www.womenshealth.gov.

9 J. R. Niebyl and M. Goodwin, "Overview of Nausea and Vomiting of Pregnancy with an Emphasis on Vitamins and Ginger," *American Journal of Obstetrics & Gynecology* 186, no. 5 (2002).

10 Romm, *The Natural.*

11 Romm, *The Natural.*

12 Romm, *The Natural.*

13 U.S. Department of Health and Human Services, "Stages of."

14 U.S. Department of Health and Human Services, "Stages of."

15 Romm, *The Natural.*

16 U.S. Department of Health and Human Services, "Stages of."

17 Johns Hopkins Medicine, "Your Pregnancy Week-by-Week," 2017, accessed March 4, 2017, https://www.hopkinsallchildrens.org/community/fit4allmoms/your-pregnancy-week-by-week.

Chapter 7

1 *Mercola*, "Two Food Additives Found to Have Estrogen-like Effects" (2009), accessed April 12, 2015. https://articles.mercola.com/sites/articles/archive/2009/03/19/two-food-additives-found-to-have-estrogenlike-effects.aspx.

2 Murray, *The Encyclopedia of Healing Foods.*

3 Murray, *The Encyclopedia of Healing Foods.*

4 Murray, *The Encyclopedia of Healing Foods.*

5   "Why Therapeutic Benefits of Coffee Do Not Apply to Pregnant Women", *Mercola*, 2014, accessed March 16, 2017, https://articles.mercola.com/sites/articles/archive/2014/02/03/coffee-in-pregnancy.aspx.

6   P. Bartholomy, Ph.D., Hawthorn University, "Life Stages and Clinical Nutrition," 2014, NC Lecture Series.

7   "No-Nonsense Guide to a Naturally Healthy Pregnancy and Baby," *Mercola*, 2009, accessed March 16, 2017, http://articles.mercola.com/sites/articles/archive/2009/11/07/.

8   *Mercola*, "No-Nonsense."

9   *Mercola*, "No-Nonsense."

10   *Mercola*, "No-Nonsense."; "Xenoestrogens."

11   Murray, *The Encyclopedia of Healing Foods*.

12   Murray, *The Encyclopedia of Healing Foods*.

13   P. Bartholomy, Ph.D., Hawthorn University, "Life Stages."

14   Romm, *The Natural*.

15   "Smoking and Fertility," accessed June 7, 2016. Yourfertility.org.au/for-men/smoking.

16   Murray, *The Encyclopedia of Healing Foods*.

17   "Smoking and Fertility."

18   "Xenoestrogens."

19   Murray, *The Encyclopedia of Natural Medicine*.

20   Murray, *The Encyclopedia of Natural Medicine*.

21   P. Bartholomy, Ph.D., "Life Stages."

22   Murray, *The Encyclopedia of Natural Medicine*.

23   P. Bartholomy, Ph.D., "Life Stages."

24   *Mercola*, "Two Food Additives."

25   *Mercola*, "Two Food Additives."

26   C. Paddock, "Women's Fertility Linked to Oral Health," *Medical News Today*, 2011, accessed March 6, 2017, www.medicalnewstoday.com/articles/230568.php.

27   *Mercola*, "No-Nonsense."

28   *Mercola*, "No-Nonsense."

Chapter 8

1 K. Laing, "How Long Does It Really Take to Recover after Pregnancy and Birth?" *Huffington Post*, August 8, 2015.

2 J. M. Miller et al., "Evaluating Maternal Recovery from Labor and Delivery: Bone and Levator Ani Injuries," *American Journal of Obstetrics & Gynecology* 203, no. 188 (2015): e1–11.

3 Miller et al., "Evaluating."

4 Laing, "How Long."

5 Laing, "How Long."

6 "Mental Health," *World Health Organization*, 2017, accessed October 1, 2016, www.who.int/mental_health/maternal-child/maternal_mental_health/en/.

7 C. Andrews-Fike, "A Review of Postpartum Depression," National Institutes of Health, *Primary Care Companion to the Journal of Clinical Psychiatry* 1, no. 1 (1999): 9–14, PMC181045.

8 S. K. Dørheim et al., "Sleep and Depression in Postpartum Women: A Population-Based Study," *Sleep* 32, no. 7 (2009): 847–855.

9 Mercola, "Postartum Depression: A Guide for New Moms," *Mercola*, 2016, accessed April 1, 2017, www.articles.mercola.com/depression/postpartum-depression.aspx.

10 S. J. Fomon, "Infant Feeding in the 20th Century: Formula and Beikost," *Journal of Nutrition* 131, no. 2 (2001): 4095–4205.

11 Fomon, "Infant Feeding."

12 Fomon, "Infant Feeding."

13 Centers for Disease Control and Prevention, "Breastfeeding Rates Continue to Rise in the U.S.," *2016 Breastfeeding Report Card*, 2017, accessed March 8, 2017, https://www.cdc.gov/breastfeeding/data/breastfeeding-report-card-2016.html.

14 Centers for Disease Control and Prevention, "Breastfeeding."

15 C. M. Dieterich et al., "Breastfeeding and Health Outcomes for the Mother-Infant Dyad," *Pediatric Clinics of North*

America 60, no. 1 (2013): 31–48, http://doi.org/10.1016/j.pcl.2012.09.010.

16 N. Butte et al., "Patient Education: Maternal Health and Nutrition during Breastfeeding (beyond the Basics)," *UpToDate.com*, 2016. Accessed June 22, 2017, https://www.uptodate.com/contents/maternal-health-and-nutrition-during-breastfeeding-beyond-the-basics?search=patient%20education:%20maternal%20health%20and%20nutrition%20during%20breastfeeding&-source=search_result&selectedTitle=1~150&usage_type=default&display_rank=1.

17 Butte et al., "Patient."

18 Butte et al., "Patient."

19 Butte et al., "Patient."

20 Haas and Levin, *Staying Healthy.*

21 B. Roehman, "Why Most Moms Don't Reach Their Own Breast-Feeding Goals," *TIME*, June 4, 2012, accessed June 22, 2017, www.healthland.time.com/2012/06/04/why-most-moms-cant-reach-their-own-breast-feeding-goals/.

22 Roehman, "Why Most."

23 Roehman, "Why Most."

24 U.S. Department of Labor, "Newborn's and Mother's Health Protection Act of 1996," accessed May 25, 2017, https://www.dol.gov/agencies/ebsa/about-ebsa/our-activities/resource-center/faqs/nmhpa.

25 Dørheim et al., "Sleep and Depression."

Chapter 9

1 U.S. Department for Health and Human Services, Centers for Disease Control and Prevention, "Dietary Supplement Use among U.S. Adults Has Increased Since NHANES III (1988–1994)," *NCHS Brief* 61 (April 2011).

2 Beatrice Tsui et al., "A Survey of Dietary Supplement Use During Pregnancy at an Academic Medical Center," *American Journal of Obstetrics & Gynecology* 185, no. 2 (2001): 433–437.

3   U.S. Department for Health and Human Services, Centers for Disease Control and Prevention, "Folic Acid Data and Statistics," 2007, accessed July 6, 2016, www.cdc.gov.ncbddd/ folicacid/data.html.

4   U.S. Department for Health and Human Services, Centers for Disease Control and Prevention, "Folic Acid."

5   C. Ulrich, "Folate and Cancer Prevention: A Closer Look at a Complex Picture," *American Journal of Clinical Nutrition* 86, no. 2 (August 2007): 271–273.

6   U.S. Department for Health and Human Services, Centers for Disease Control and Prevention, "Folic Acid.

7   U.S. Department for Health and Human Services, Centers for Disease Control and Prevention, "Overweight & Obesity," 2014, accessed July 6, 2016, https://www.cdc.gov/obesity/data/ adult.html.

8   Epp Davis and H. D. Riordan, "Changes in USDA Food Composition Data for 43 Garden Crops, 1950 to 1999," *Journal of the American College of Nutrition* 23, no. 6 (December 2004): 669–682.

9   "Weston A. Price, DDS," *Weston A. Price Foundation,* 2000, accessed July 6, 2016, www.westonaprice.org/health-topics/ weston-a-price-dds/.

10   Nasdaq Globe Newswire, "Dietary Supplements Market Size," *Grand View Research, Inc.*, July 2016, accessed March 2, 2017, https://globenewswire.com/ news-release/2016/07/18/856668/0/en/.

11   U.S. Department of Health and Human Services, FDA, "Current Good Manufacturing Practice in Manufacturing, Packaging, Labeling or Holding Operations for Dietary Supplements; Small Entity Compliance Guide," accessed August 12, 2016, www.fda. gov/food/guidanceregulation/guidancedocumentsregulatoryinfor- mation/DietarySupplements/ucm238182.htm.

12   "About NPA," *Natural Products Association (NPA)*, 2016, accessed August 12, 2016, www.npainfo.org/NPA/About_NPA/History/ NPA/AboutNPA/History.aspx.

13   "About NPA."

14   A. W. Saul, "Orthomolecular Medicine on the Internet," *Journal of Orthomolecular Medicine* 20, no. 2 (2005), www.orthomolecular.org/library/jom/2005/pdf/2005-v20n02-p070.pdf.

15   U.S. Department of Health and Human Services, FDA, "Current Good."; "The Doctor Oz Show: Information I Couldn't Share," Mercola, 2014, accessed August 12, 2016, www.articles.mercola.com/sites/articles/archive/2014/02/06/supplements-safety-issues.aspx.

16   Hawthorn University, "Selecting High Quality Dietary Supplements—Finding the Products and Companies You Can Trust," 2010, accessed August 12, 2016, www.portal.hawthornuniversity.org/course_readingmateriallist.aspx.

17   Kedar N. Prasad, *Vitamins in Cancer Prevention and Treatment* (Rochester, Vermont: Healing Arts Press, 1994).

18   Hawthorn University, "Selecting High."

19   Hawthorn University, "Selecting High."

Appendix

1   "Food Sources of Potassium," *Organix*, formerly Epigenetic Labs, 2017, accessed June 1, 2017. https://organix.com.

2   Mateljan, *The World's*.

3   Haas and Levin, *Staying Healthy*.

4   J. Krone and F. Taylor, *Natural Detoxification, 2nd Edition* (Vancouver: Hartley & Marks Publishers, Inc., 2000).

5   Rebekah Fedrowitz, "Antioxidant Salad," *You Are Well Health*, 2017, www.youarewellhealth.com.

6   Mateljan, *The World's*.

ACKNOWLEDGMENTS

This is my first book. Writing and publishing it has given me a new sense of clarity and insight as to why authors consider each book a labor of love. It is a time-consuming, arduous task that requires passion, patience, and determination to see through to completion. In addition to the years I spent organizing and writing the content, getting to the final product truly took a village of experts to design, edit, and market the final copy.

To my "village" I offer my most heartfelt gratitude: Debby Englander, my publishing consultant, Ramona Richards, whose expertise was invaluable with technical editing, my daughter Becky Ingram, who helped me navigate the world of social media, and the very professional, talented team at Post Hill Press. Collectively, you helped turn my thoughts and message into a resource that offers hope to many who dream of becoming parents.

I will always be grateful for the unending encouragement, patience, and support I received from my immediate family and closest friends (you know who you are). The attention I gave to writing and researching this book over three-plus years often meant not spending time with all of you. I am so fortunate to have each and every one of you in my life.

ABOUT THE AUTHOR

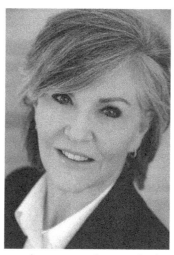

After a five-and-a-half-year-long battle with MS, Barbara Rodgers used holistic nutrition protocols to heal herself from this devastating disease. She was inspired to return to school to study Holistic Nutrition, and is now a Nutrition Consultant; board certified in Holistic Nutrition. Barbara helps individuals with chronic disease, unexplained infertility, and autoimmune conditions understand the effect their diet and lifestyle choices have as contributing factors to overall health.

After twenty-six years of experience working in corporate America, Barbara effectively taps into her well-honed business acumen and relationship skills when working with clients to develop customized nutrition strategies. Positions formerly held include senior vice president and national sales manager for Fiserv Securities in Philadelphia, PA, and Director, Global Clients for SunGard in New York. Barbara is currently an executive board member of the National Association of Nutrition Professionals (NANP) and resides in Philadelphia, PA, where she works virtually with clients across the U.S.

For more information, visit www.nutritionlifestrategies.com